FAT
KIDS

FAT KIDS

Truth and Consequences

REBECCA JANE WEINSTEIN

BEAUFORT
BOOKS

BEAUFORT BOOKS
NEW YORK

Library of Congress Cataloging-in-Publication Data

Weinstein, Rebecca Jane, 1967-
Fat kids : truth and consequences / by Rebecca Jane Weinstein. -- First edition.
pages cm
Includes bibliographical references and index.
ISBN 978-0-8253-0725-6 (hardcover : alk. paper)
1. Obesity in children. 2. Body image in children. I. Title.
RJ399.C6W447 2014
618.92'398--dc23
2014016242

For inquiries about volume orders, please contact:

Beaufort Books
27 West 20th Street, Suite 1102
New York, NY 10011
sales@beaufortbooks.com

Published in the United States by Beaufort Books
www.beaufortbooks.com

Distributed by Midpoint Trade Books
www.midpointtrade.com

Printed in the United States of America

Interior design by Jamie Kerry of Belle Étoile Studios
Cover Design by Michael Short

FAT
KIDS

This book is dedicated to all the fat kids, former fat kids, and kids who think they are fat.

CONTENTS

PART THREE

PART FOUR

ACKNOWLEDGMENTS

Without the contributions and support from the following individuals, this book would not have been written: my parents, Joyce Ellen Weinstein and Mark Weinstein; Michael Wright of Garson & Wright Public Relations; everyone at Beaufort Books; my friend and editor, Buffy Morrissette; Becky McKinnell of iBec Creative; contributors Nikki Blonsky, Pattie Thomas, Peggy Elam, Sarah Yahm, Emily Dhurandhar, and Daniel Pinkwater; also Theresa Dyer Bakker, Patricia Washburn, Cheryl Fuller, Cassandra Lupi, and Mark Ebner; and everyone who shared their illuminating and very personal stories. Thank you.

Thank you also to the supporters of this book: Howard Glickberg, Susan Stearns, Terri Weitze, Lily O'Hara, Chris Bentley, BBWGeneration, Barbara Shapiro, Leanne Dempsey, Buffy Joseph, Bri King, Homalyn Krakowski, Lizbeth Binks Carney, Tegan E. Stover, Shannon Halvorsen, Michelle Wilkinson, Holin Fung, Pamela Punger, Brenda Oelbaum, Dayna M. Reidenouer, Joan Reilly, Bernd Zetsche, Kerry A. Beake, Lara Frater, Ariane Blanch, Sarah Smith, Celine Stillman, Danielle Agape Biconik, Jennifer Weigel, Deb Lemire, T. A. Spackman, Diana Johns, Mandy Wheeler, Jennifer E. Levine, Kristen Dunn, Gayle Lin, Liz Cutler, Judith Matz, Jaime Bolland, Kennon Hulett, Deb Burgard, Dennis Burger, LargeInCharge.com, Kevin J. Maroney, Marie Merillat, Robin Wheeler, Kathy Kater, Emily Philp, Christopher Martin, Kate Ahern, Mike Coulter, Tom Naughton, Sarah Jessica Farber, Brigid Hagan, Lesleigh Owen, Jenny Jameson, Ben G. Mandall,

Wednesday Lee Friday, Jessica Brown, Robynne Blumë, Shannon O'Leary, Joan Reilly, Lauren Collins, Jeliza Patterson, Kalamity Hildebrandt, Valerie X. Armstrong, Stephanie Wichmann, Tamara Pincus, Louise Larsen, Helen Honey, Amy Dobek, Caitlin Holland, Marsi Burns, Lisa Kasen, Miriam Gordon, Julia Starkey, Bobbie-Jo Elwood, Julie Voit Levinson, Jennifer Jonassen, Lori Watts.

INTRODUCTION

Fat Kids: Truth and Consequences tells the real-life stories behind being a fat kid. At this critical juncture, kids are struggling—fat kids, skinny kids, girl kids, and boy kids. The pressure to be thin is overwhelming. The devastation that is happening to kids because of weight, bullying, shame, fear, pills, surgeries, and profound pain is ever-growing. The childhood obesity crisis around the world may be troubling, but there are other reasons for concern besides fat kids. And everyone—kids, their parents, and all the well-meaning people trying to protect these kids from their fat bodies—needs to know the truth and consequences. We must not focus only on their fat; we must protect kids' hearts, souls, and sanity as well. These are stories of fat kids, former fat kids, and kids who think they are fat. Their stories need to be told. They will make you cry, and then they will make you think.

Whether we call it an "epidemic" or a "war," children are in the midst of a battle for their lives, for their physical, emotional, and social existence. As fat kids, those who are perceived as such or even just those who simply feel fat, children, as they grow into teenagers and adults, are struggling in ways more profound than the media or even the medical establishment would lead us to believe. And it's not primarily because of deadly pounds; the issues are far more complex than that. Although discussion is at a fever pitch now, it has been decades in the making. There is nothing new about children on diets, children on diet pills, children in intense weight-loss programs such as camps and schools. But now it is in the news, and the message is one of life and death.

Whether that message leads to weight loss, lifestyle changes, responses from the food industry, and happier, healthier children is certainly unclear. In fact it is so unclear, the truth and consequences are rarely discussed. What is even more hidden is the struggle, often lifelong, that is burdening these children. From shame to bullying, from eating disorders to feelings of self-defeat and lack of self-esteem, and all of the emotional and physical costs of what is so often a frustrating and even futile battle, fat kids are impacted by being fat, and by the expectation of becoming thin, in ways most people cannot comprehend.

It is time their stories are told.

This book is an account of people's real life experiences growing up fat and being the parents of fat children, the methods that were used to cause weight loss, and the outcomes of these experiences. Heartfelt and often heartbreaking real-life stories are paired with expert discussion of important issues of the day, such as stigma and bullying, the psychological ramifications of being a fat child in our culture, and the medical science behind weight. This book includes honest and forthright portrayals in a memoir-esque storytelling style, used to illustrate the serious information presented by subject-matter experts.

These accounts, while anecdotal, are a good representation of varied life experiences. Interviewees were not cherry-picked but rather volunteered after learning of the interviews in notices available to the public. The author does not personally know any of these people. The interviews were open-ended, with people discussing the issues they felt most important to them. Whether one agrees or disagrees with any particular perspective, these are true, heartfelt stories, often told through tears, and often for the very first time.

The value of the experience of this book, for the participants, the author, and potentially the public, cannot be overstated, nor can the gratitude felt for everyone involved, for their courage, generosity, and open hearts.

PART ONE

PROLOGUE

A TASTE OF BITTER

I remember that red lollipop like I wasn't six years old then and forty-six now. Before being bestowed that glistening cellophane-wrapped, ruby-red, cherry-sweet consolation prize, I was just a little kid trapped in a world of grown-ups who hated themselves for reasons they were too ill-equipped to identify. After, I served a very important role. I was broken, and everyone's identified project to fix. I was finally needed.

Oh, everyone had good intentions. There is certainly nothing more honorable than to repair a damaged child. But we all know what the road to hell is paved with, and as the doctor held up that sugary treat—the apparent reward for being a child, despite my pending punishment for my flawed job at being one—I was set squarely on the pavement.

The story goes more or less like this: My parents were hippies, artists, and freaks. They should never have been married, but they were, and they should never have had children, but they did, and during the prolonged collapse of the partnership, perhaps I was soothed with the only drug-like substance you can give a child. Or my mother started me on rice too early. Or nobody did anything wrong and my body just happened to be larger than was fashionable in the early 1970s.

My mother's relatives, wealthy and self-important, had me seen by the "best" pediatrician in New York City. You can't scrimp on a child's medical care. At my sixth birthday checkup, I was found to be at the top of the percentile chart for fatness in children, and I was prescribed a diet. Then I was given the red lollipop. A child's first irony. Don't think I didn't notice.

As explained to me decades later, no one gave my parents instruction on putting a six-year-old on a diet. Parents like mine didn't ask questions, and doctors like mine didn't offer explanations. I don't actually recall what being on a diet as a six-year-old was like. But I do recall that my mother told my first-grade teacher I was on one. My teacher was, in my recollection, a sadist, and she brought me to the front of the room and informed the class that she and I were both on a diet, so we wouldn't be having birthday cake with the rest of the class.

If you think I didn't catch the import of this little performance, you would be wrong. Two years later, my brother was in her class. I was in the third grade and a slew of kids came down with lice. Rumor had it Mrs. Silverstein said my brother was infected with the dirty, dirty lice. I still harbored such a grudge from my prior humiliation that I called her a "lying bitch." When you are eight and it's 1975, that is serious smack talk. Someone squealed, and my third-grade butt was hauled down to her classroom so that I could apologize to her in person, in front of the class. I don't remember what exactly I was made to apologize for. It's doubtful I announced to the first graders that I was deeply sorry I called Mrs. Silverstein a lying bitch. But I do remember being in front of that room, once again.

I suppose, as it turns out, Mrs. Silverstein wasn't a liar—my brother did have lice—but she certainly was a sadist. I know that for a fact. Even a third grader is old enough to know a sadist when she has been affronted by one. Or, at least, that's how I remember it—maybe I'm projecting a bit, but this kind of thing scars a person for life. Mrs. Silverstein is probably dead now. She seemed really, really old when I knew her. Regardless, I had my fingers crossed when I apologized, but even if I didn't, I wasn't sorry then, and I'm not sorry now.

Standardized government height and weight charts, or "growth charts," to establish whether a child is in "normal" range, were not developed until 1977. The Centers for Disease Control and Prevention (CDC) developed these charts, using data that had been collected since the 1960s, to determine if a child's growth was sufficient—if a child had grown enough to meet health standards. The World Health Organization also adopted these CDC charts for international use. In 2000, these charts were updated to account for more diverse populations and the differences between breast-fed and bottle-fed children, breast-fed tending to be larger. After a 1997 "expert committee on the assessment and treatment of childhood obesity" concluded that body mass index (BMI) should be used to screen for overweight children, a BMI measurement was included for children ages two years and older. BMI (weight (lb) / [height (in)]2 x 703) is calculated from weight and height measurements and is used to judge whether an individual's weight is appropriate for their height.

Before that, whether a child was too thin or too fat was a matter of individual assessment. Did the kid appear too thin or too fat? And the concern was primarily whether the kid was too thin. Too fat wasn't generally an issue in young children. Weighing children became popular around 1910 when public health workers aimed to identify those who were malnourished. Widespread malnutrition was declared after tens of thousands of children were weighed in schools, church basements, and public facilities. A decade later, doctors concluded that weight was not sufficient alone to identify malnutrition and that a full examination and medical history were needed. By the 1930s, weight charts were just one tool used for measuring the health of children, now determined in a doctor's office. Still, fat children were hardly the primary concern.

I was declared too fat in 1973, before government charts. Unlike my parents' generation—children during the Second World War and right after the Great Depression, during which time doctors would likely have been pleased to find a child in the top percentile—I was examined at the tail end of Twiggy's swinging

'60s. The curvaceous bombshells such as Mae West, Jane Russell, and Marilyn Monroe, were out, and the androgynous, waif-like Twiggy, Edie Sedgwick, and Mia Farrow were in.

That's not to say there wasn't a precursor to this look during Marilyn's day. In the 1950s and even a century before, gamine women—slim, boyish, wide-eyed, and perceived as mischievous and teasing—had their place in ideal beauty: Audrey Hepburn, and before her, Mary Pickford and Lillian Gish. But this look—the gamine, before the '60s waif—was an exception, not the rule. It wasn't until the sexual revolution that androgyny took a real hold on American culture. And when it did take hold, it held on hard. Later called *heroin chic*, and now just *fashion-model thin*, it has been *a* predominant ideal, if not *the* predominant ideal, ever since. Today there is great debate whenever a woman in the public eye is more buxom. Is she voluptuous or fat? And this pervasive discussion filters into every aspect of society, including the medical profession, and certainly the social worlds of young girls.

At any rate, being born at the height of the sexual revolution and the waif period, mine was perhaps the first generation of children, particularly girls, who were singled out for being fat as young children. Prepubescent, preadolescent children. This was well before fast-food was ubiquitous. Processed food was in its infancy. Meals were sit-down. Soda, cake, and candy were still for special occasions. Nonetheless, thin was in. So chubby at six, I was put on a diet. Diets were also in. In fact, perhaps a peculiar corollary to the sexual revolution was the mass diet industry. Women were dieting. Mothers were dieting. So for the first time, it was conceivable that little girls could diet along, too.

To the best of my knowledge my mother wasn't a dieter. She did think she was fat and it was always an issue for her. I believe she avoided certain foods, but I don't recall that she joined me in any formal plan. I was the sole dieter in the family. Six, seven, eight, nine, and so forth, I dieted. I dieted every day of my childhood. Or at least I was supposed to be dieting, and I was monitored closely. So I had to learn the tricks of the trade early on, which I did.

For some reason there was a lot of cheese involved. What *diet* ended up meaning, in not too short an order, was a battle of the wills. My mother put me on a diet, and I put me on a mission to eat whatever I could without getting caught. I don't remember if I was hungry or if I did whatever I could to acquire food on principle. But I ate a lot of the Weight Watchers treats that involved putting cottage cheese, saccharine, and cinnamon on low-calorie bread, which was then baked to vaguely resemble (or be an illusion of resemblance to) some kind of cheese-cake-type-facsimile concoction. I can still taste that in my memory now. It's not even that they tasted terrible, which they did, but they seemed terrible, which they were.

My house was a no-junk-food zone. Which also meant no sugar or nondiet desserts. There wasn't a whole lot of junk food to speak of back then, so "no junk food" probably isn't accurate. It was a no-fat-people-food zone. Except I was the only fat person, so my brother, skinny as a rail, would get different foods. He would get "treats," but also just nondietetic consumables. It's fairly vague, but some of the food was my brother's, and some was mine. There were also stores of sweets hidden very high in cupboards that I didn't know about, except I knew about them. I was good at climbing for a fat kid.

But what I remember the most was cheese. Cheddar cheese. There was always a block of cheddar cheese in the fridge. My job, as I saw it, was to eat as much cheddar cheese as I could without raising suspicion. This meant both being very quiet and also somehow making the cheese appear as if it hadn't been violated. I doubt very seriously I accomplished either of those goals, but my mother's apathy allowed me to complete the caper frequently.

I did get caught on occasion. My mother enjoyed a good sting operation. In fact, shock and awe was her favorite tactical maneuver. My brother and I walked to elementary school, and on the way was a newsstand that sold this and that. My brother would get a quarter (perhaps it was a dime) to buy a banana for a snack. He was in kindergarten or first grade, which meant I was in second or third. It was not terribly hard to convince him to buy penny candy with the money instead, which we did on a regular basis. Now, frankly, if children our age didn't buy penny candy instead of a banana with the quarter (or dime), there would have been something else suspicious going on. But in our household, this was a major crime. A tactical team was employed. My mother and her best friend, our next-door neighbor (a social worker for Christ's sake), tracked us using the most sophisticated technology. They followed us to school, walking across the street and several feet behind. Witnessing the transaction at the newsstand, they had all the evidence they needed for the bust. They waited for maximum impact, and when we got to the schoolyard, a good six blocks farther, I was confronted. They let the innocent go. My brother was set free. Only I was held captive, and for my crime I was interrogated using the most brutal and heinous of strategies: I was asked in front of my friends, "Isn't it true you purchased candy with your brother's banana money?" The light was so bright shining in my eyes. Next was waterboarding, I knew it. I had no choice but to lie. "No." But the jig was up. It was bananas from then on. What they didn't know, these captors, the enemy, the assassins, was I still had my cheddar cheese. *Viva la revolución!*

There are endless stories I can tell about my escapades as a dieting child. Wacky stuff. Like the time I blamed my little brother for eating all the special sugar cereal (this was at my dad's; there, sugar cereal was legal on the Fourth of July and presidential birthdays). I still remember the inquisition. It was more preposterous that I blamed my brother for that than for forgoing the banana. Luckily my father had a smaller army and my punishment was less severe—only private humiliation. The truth was, there was no division of food at my father's house. He was the first, and only, person to let me eat a McDonald's cheeseburger as a child. But compulsion knows no address. Once I learned I needed to steal food to eat, it was difficult to remember where that applied, and where it didn't. I was just a kid. I mean, I was just a kid.

I learned where the food was, which of my friends' houses were well stocked and which parents had an open bar. When I got a little older, but not much older, and could go out to stores on my own, where there was little parental supervision beyond that of food monitor, I found what could be bought and eaten during any given surreptitious errand.

The long and the short of it is I was not so much put on a diet at six, as much as given the eating-disorder starter package. Not to mention the initiation into the society for lying and mistrust.

As the story goes, I didn't get "really fat" until I was sent to Girl Scout camp one summer. I was about eleven. It was the year before fat camp. While there, I was tortured by the girls in my bunk. I don't say "tortured" lightly. When I would walk by them they would chant in unison, "Here comes the tub." I assure you that still rings loudly in my head. Because that camp was not built to protect fat kids from themselves; food was plentiful, and there wasn't much comfort for me in anything else. Although I can't say it was only comfort I was looking for. I had never been able to just eat what I had wanted before, and that part of camp was fun. Toward the end of camp, I had some kind of mental breakdown, or so they thought. I spent at least a week in the infirmary, where they threatened that if I didn't get better, they wouldn't let me go home. I magically got better—proving, of course, that I was simply neurotic, and that I could be threatened out of it.

Here's the thing, though. The infirmary wasn't exactly the Mayo Clinic, and while lying in my infirmary bed, I found this thing attached to my head. It seemed really big, and it was squishy. I spent days trying to pick it off from under my hair. I thought I had a tumor and that I could remove it by picking at it (I was eleven). I was kind of right. I accomplished the extraction and found in my hand this bloody glob. It creeped the hell out of me and I threw it under the next bed. It was years later that I realized it was an engorged tick. Fancy that, I was actually sick, but too afraid to tell anyone about this growth. I didn't magically get better. I performed minor surgery on myself and was no longer a host to a predator. I left camp fatter, now a mental case, and so ashamed that no one ever knew about the tick. To this day, only a few people know, until now.

The next summer, and the summer after that, I was sent to fat camp. I came home from junior high one day, and my mother, loving the element of surprise as she did, had a pile of fat-camp brochures as high as an elephant's eye. There was a big fight. I lost. I went to fat camp, which, frankly, I enjoyed. I was just one of them there, although there was still a hierarchy. The thinner kids were the better kids (they just weren't as thin as the better kids at home). I lost a lot of weight, two summers in a row, and by high school I was sort of normal. Now, maintaining that normal was something else.

Throughout high school I learned about speed and compulsive exercise, and a good friend taught me about laxatives. She warned me: "Never take these." So of course I bought the family-size box. I managed to stay a normalish weight throughout high school, but only with the assistance of well-honed eating disorders and copious amounts of self-loathing. My father once said I was lucky to have the eating disorder because my mother had plans for me to undergo weight-loss surgery, and I was saved from internal mutilation by emotional wreckage. My mother's recollection is different, and I'll give her the benefit of the doubt, but at the time if she had wanted me to have weight-loss surgery, I probably would have thought the idea brilliant.

Then I went to college, where, of course, there were no food police, and I gained weight. I lost weight. I gained weight. I grew up. I lost weight. I gained weight. Ultimately I spent decades weighing somewhere between 250 and 350 pounds. I did a ton of therapy, including treatment for PTSD, and forty years after my first diet I seem to be eating-disorder free. I don't know what I weigh. I have joined the ranks of the "size acceptance movement," though I wouldn't say I am a card-carrying member. I certainly believe in social justice for fat people, that the multibillion-dollar diet industry is corrupt, that the focus should be on good health and not low weight, and that hating oneself serves no productive purpose whatsoever. Mostly, I am in it for the emotional healing, and it has helped. I also write about fat. That helps, when it doesn't rip my heart to shreds.

I am certainly not a "happy-go-lucky" person, but that may be partially my inborn personality. I am also as bitter as I sound, sometimes. But I have a good sense of humor and this has been my burden, which made me strong and relentless. And while I would change everything, I try to appreciate what I have learned. The best thing that has happened from all this is I stood up to my parents, over the course of a decade, and taught them they needed to love me the way I am—and they do. This experience has made us all better people. They support my work, in more ways than one, and I have seen proof positive that people can change, dramatically. I am cautiously optimistic the second half of my life will be easier, and happier, and will last as long as the first.

I am grateful for what I can be grateful for, and have some rational understanding of what used to seem like pure insanity. I know children should not be put on diets as I was, and I present their stories because I am tired of fat people, and especially fat children, being misunderstood, and paying the price for that misunderstanding. Clearly, working to that end is what I was built for, whether I like it or not.

That's my story, and I'm stuck with it.

1

WHO'S THE FAT COW NOW?

Ethnographic Insights on the Academy of the Sierras

BY SARAH YAHM

Wellspring Academy of California, the first therapeutic weight-loss boarding school for obese and overweight teens, is a series of squat, low-slung red bungalows surrounded by miles of Sun-Maid raisin fields.[1] You might have heard of them, either from their feature in the *New York Times* or their *Dateline* special, or maybe you've watched their reality TV show, *Too Fat for 15*, set on their North Carolina campus.

In the fall of 2007, when I showed up with my microphone, they'd only been in business for three years, but they'd already garnered a seemingly endless series of positive press coverage. I'd called their press officer the week before, explaining that I was a graduate student creating a series of audio documentaries about the obesity epidemic. I was surprised when he responded so quickly and positively to my request for a visit, since schools usually zealously guard their students' privacy.

Sure I could come, he told me, and yes it was fine for me to bring my microphone; all of the parents signed release forms for

---

1   In April 2008, Academy of the Sierras changed its name to Wellspring Academy of California.

their kids with their admissions paperwork. In retrospect, it's not surprising at all, considering they created *Too Fat for 15* just a few years later, which publicly features the transformation of fat kids from "freaks" to productive citizens. Their goal is not just to "cure" the kids in their care, but also to spread their "healthy obsession" doctrine into the belly of the beast itself, America's obesogenic society.

When the woman working the motel desk in Reedley, California, hears that I am a reporter going to the academy she leans forward conspiratorially, even though there is no one else in the room, and says, "They should really investigate that place." And then she nods meaningfully and gives me the dirt. Apparently all of the parents stay there the night before they drop off their kids. Some of them, she says, are filthy rich—"you can tell from the way they talk to you"—but others don't have that much money. "Some people," she says, "have second or third mortgages on their home to pay for the tuition. And some of the kids," she continues, winding herself up, "aren't even fat." She points down at her own belly. "I know fat," she says. "And they're not fat."

I nod because I also know fat, but the more I do my research the less I seem to understand it. Wellspring was not the first step on my fat research tour—I'd already hung out with fat activists in New York and San Francisco and interviewed Christian dieters in the Central Valley in California. By the time I arrived at Wellspring, I had no idea if I was skinny or fat—I was living in my own personal *Alice in Wonderland*. When I interviewed fat activists, I felt skinny; when I interviewed dieters, I felt fat. In the span of one subway ride, I would shrink and grow, shrink and grow, until I had no perspective anymore on anyone's size, including my own. And the more I researched it, the less I seemed to care who was fat and who wasn't. The point of fat, I'd concluded, was that it had no point, which was why I was so frightened about the idea of a school predicated entirely upon eliminating it.

When I arrive on campus the next morning, the woman at the front desk directs me to the behavioral coach's office. I apologize for making her walk me there, and she says, "Oh, don't worry about it. It'll help me get in my ten thousand steps." Apparently, all of the staff are required to self-monitor, not just the kids. And they (the almost entirely skinny and fit staff) do it gleefully, writing in their self-monitoring journals and wearing their pedometers with pride. Weight loss, they explain, is a community effort. And we all need to learn to self-monitor. The behavioral coach, a fit young twentysomething, expands upon this idea as soon as we're seated in her cramped office in the main bungalow. "Everybody could self-monitor," she explains. "Everybody should. Everybody should be; ideally, that's what we expect." As she talks about Dr. Kirschenbaum, their founder, and the premise of "the healthy obsession," it dawns on me that she's not really talking about fat kids at all; she's talking about a philosophy of life. "What we want," she explains, "is to have these kids become obsessed with being a weight-controller. That's what we know works over time.... What we know is that the kids who are successful when they leave here are the kids who are obsessed with getting ten thousand steps a day. We have kids who've been at nine thousand something and will walk around their living room to make sure they get the ten thousand steps a day."

I interrupt her because as the daughter of two psychoanalysts and a veteran of a fair amount of therapy myself, the notion of a healthy obsession is a bit hard to swallow. She is undeterred: "As I said before, there's nothing convenient about being a weight-controller, so it really does take that amount of commitment and obsessive approach to really getting it done and really doing it, but it's completely doable. So, to answer your question in a more broad sense, the obsessive quality about it is what works, and part of why we have the clinical program and therapeutic program with it is to turn any kind of obsessive thinking into something that's healthy. Ideally you want someone who is very detail-oriented and is very meticulous in their self-monitoring, very accurate and things like that."

* * *

Of course, having been a chubby kid growing up in the United States, I know that living with this type of obsession is completely doable. I've seen most of my friends do it. I've also seen them go through treatment for years to learn how to stop doing it. The question that I don't ask the behavioral coach, but I do ask the kids, is *why* do it? They give me a couple of reasons: "So I don't die when I'm twenty." "To get healthier." "It's important to my mom, to be healthy." Throughout it all looms the unquestioned threat of imminent death—the kids talk as if Wellspring is single-handedly snatching them from its jaws. But when they're pressed they reveal an aching desire that has nothing to do with health and everything to do with being normal:

"It's gonna mess with my brain enough so I'll stay with my program after nine months and be hopefully normal."

"I wanna be skinny; I love fitting into clothes. I used to be skinny and I want to be skinny again."

"I don't know if people are gonna, like, change the way they act towards me but I'm looking forward to coming home, and this one boy called me a fat cow and I'm just gonna go up to him and be like, 'Who's the fat cow now?' because he's like heavy and he got really heavy over the summer, and he was so mean to me, so I'm just gonna go up to him and be like, 'Hi.'"

One kid even tells me that "fatties" should be picked on more, that society is too accepting of fat kids, that maybe taunting helps kids decide that "Oh, well maybe I don't want to be a fatty anymore." The overarching lesson they're learning is quite clear—deviance should be punished, and the only way to be happy is to stop being deviant. Losing weight is about being cool, about having friends, about winning their parents' approval, about not being picked on.

* * *

After talking to the behavioral coach and the headmaster, they let me loose with my microphone, confident that the success of the place speaks for itself. Over my two visits, I walk the morning walk with a group of kids, I attend a school-wide meeting where kids are allotted special privileges based on how well they self-monitor, I mill around during the post-weigh-in chaos, I interview individual students, and I hang out in the cafeteria with a group of disgruntled teenage boys. By the end of my visits, I have a very clear sense of how the healthy obsession works and the costs that it requires.

The heart of the Wellspring experience (and the subsequent TV show, *Too Fat for 15*) is the scale, which looms over the daily lives of students. It is the only valid unit of measure. For instance, a student, let's call him Henry, who did a triathlon over the weekend but only lost 2 pounds has a sense of failure, not a sense of accomplishment. I meet up with Henry, my tour guide for the day, on the lawn just after the weigh-in ritual. The students are milling about comparing weights like scores on a math quiz. A girl runs over to us to share her good news.

"I lost seven!"

"You lost seven?" Henry looks visibly upset. "I hate you!"

"How'd you do?" she asks him.

"I only lost two." He drops his head and shuffles his feet, looking ashamed.

"That's good, that's *good*! At least you're losing," she says in a chipper, enthusiastic tone.

Wellspring emphasizes the supportive community among students, although this encouragement barely disguises a panicked competition. Henry begins to frantically do math out loud.

"My first week here I lost 16, and I usually average about 5 pounds, right? I mean 82 pounds in 13 weeks, that's more than 2 pounds a week." He trails off and his friend changes the topic.

"Oh, by the way, I get my cartilage pierced 'cause I'm at the 56-pound mark, when I hit 50 my mom said I could get my cartilage pierced."

"Fifty-six pounds?" Henry asks.

They continue to chat, but Henry is clearly distracted. Later, he confesses to me in private that he's very upset about his weigh-in today, and that he thinks it's because of the number of calories he ate during his triathlon. "It's one of my lowest since I got here, and I try and set goals for myself, numbers to reach. On Sunday [the day of the triathlon], when I had so many calories, I just didn't know what to do, and I was pretty upset with myself."

Henry is the model of the healthy obsession. He not only self-monitors obsessively but he also takes pleasure in it. "It's just so *fun*," he tells me unself-consciously. "I love it so much because I love seeing exactly how much I've eaten this week. And it's a really good way to stop and notice how much you're eating and sometimes it might honestly prevent you from eating something more than you should because you think, 'I have to self-monitor that, and I have to live with the fact that I ate that.'"

Clearly, losing 16 pounds a week and eating fewer than ten grams of fat a day is not and cannot be healthy, especially when large amounts of exercise are required. During an interview with a former Wellspring parent, she explained the damaging and on-going aftereffects of the "healthy obsession" model. "What I saw my daughter do, and what she said a lot of the other kids did, was obsess too much and cut out too many things, and it was an unhealthy obsession." She spoke to me from her home under the condition of anonymity because she was afraid of Wellspring's legal team. "They're cutting out too many calories and not getting enough grams of fat in their diet. What concerned me was that they were switching one eating disorder for another. She was afraid to eat, she wouldn't eat anything with fat in it; she was eating 700 to 900 calories a day. She was sick, she had gallstones, ended up having pancreatitis from her gallstones. She had to get through that and learn that she could eat things, that her body needed to have some fat in it."

Being a long-term weight-controller may in the end mean being skinnier, or it may not. The biology of fat is intricate and complicated. But it does mean living a life of ongoing punishing self-regulation. The question is do we want our kids to attempt to live their lives trying to be "long-term weight-controllers," or do we want them, simply, to live their lives unencumbered by anxiety. Henry may be "healthier" according to the scale, but he's leaving Wellspring with an obsession that's remarkably unhealthy, and a commitment to maintaining that obsession in perpetuity.

On my last day, right before I left, I walked up to a student who was sitting under a tree quietly reading a book by Toni Morrison. She bemoaned the fact that Wellspring doesn't have a library and that she has to get her parents to ship her books all the way out from the East Coast. Yes, she concedes, she's skinnier since she's been at Wellspring, but she hasn't really learned anything. She put down her book and looked at me. "Skinny is great," she said, "but, I don't want to be remembered for being skinny."

Sarah Yahm is a PhD student in American Studies at Brown University, a freelance audio producer, and an educator. This written piece emerged from her audio MA thesis produced for the Social Documentation program at the University of California, Santa Cruz. Her documentary work has appeared on transom.org, thirdcoastfestival.org, The California Report from KQED, UnFictional from KCRW, and a variety of NPR stations around the country.

2

THE MAMAS

Dr. Ivy is, among other things, an actress and a therapist. She is also a fat child, a fat mother, a fat daughter, a fat relative, and a relative of fat people. Fat runs in her family, and in many respects, ran her family. Though to be more accurate, it wasn't so much the fat that ran the family as the desperate need to be rid of it. She comes from a family where the inability to lose fat overshadowed nearly everything else anyone gained, including fame, fortune, and public admiration. Fat equaled failure, despite all evidence to the contrary.

Though Ivy works professionally with people who have eating disorders and body-image issues similar to those she experienced herself and overcame, the most important work she has performed is undoubtedly being the mother of a fat child. Therapist is one thing, mother is another. Having been a fat child herself, she especially knows the damage that can be done when raising a fat kid goes wrong.

To be perfectly honest, which is not always easy to do, when Ivy found out she was pregnant with a boy her first reaction was relief. She figured a boy wouldn't go through the same angst if he turned out to be short and round, like her. She figured there was more latitude for boys than girls, and even if he didn't turn out to be an Adonis, no one would tell a boy that his fat ass was reason enough to be unloved. That was Ivy's experience as a child: She was expected to hate herself, and logically others would follow. If your ass doesn't fit in, neither does the rest of you. Ivy's ass never fit in. Following Ivy's relief, she felt guilt. But a little guilt is better than a lifetime of worry. Protecting a fat girl was a whole different ball game than protecting a fat boy, even at ball games.

As fate, or maybe just genetics, would have it, Ivy's son did resemble his mother. And though she suspects he did get spared some of the humiliation the world inflicts on a fat girl, he wasn't entirely untouched. He was teased for being short and round. Although given the ingrained protections that Ivy ensured he had, such behavior was more of a curiosity than a catastrophe. Ivy probably could have handled a girl.

In their best attempt to disgrace him, his school chums identified him as the Pillsbury Doughboy. Certainly, we all understand the reference, but the negative implication led more to cognitive dissonance than emotional turmoil. To her son, the Pillsbury Doughboy was cute, snuggly, giggly, lovable, and associated with yummy treats. Though he understood the intent of the nickname, this really was a case of sticks and stones. He wasn't thrilled about being teased, of course, but it didn't cut through his heart like a knife into a tender biscuit. Words don't break your bones, if you aren't already fractured.

Though her son handled the mocking well, it wasn't as if he was born (even as a boy) invulnerable to feeling insecure. To combat that was work—mostly for Ivy. She felt it was challenging for a parent to help a kid maintain good self-esteem when messages from the outside world were so negative. An understatement on her part, no doubt.

He was an active child. He played softball and was in Little League, and he ran everywhere. He was not a sit-in-front-of-the-TV kind of guy. He was round because, well, he was. This was difficult for him to understand—why could his friends eat cake and ice cream, French fries and French toast, and stay slim? And more important, why didn't they get a quizzical look when asking for seconds? There was only so much Ivy could do to protect him from the judgment of others. His grandparents, aunts and uncles, and random people who had even less of a right to an opinion, managed to find a way to let him know what fat people should, and shouldn't, do. It was difficult for him to know whom to believe. His mom assured him he was just fine the way he was. She was concerned only about his health, which was also just fine. And she cared that he felt good about himself, was happy, participated in the world, and understood that not everyone looked the same. This was a conflict, particularly when well-meaning people would console him that he would surely thin out when he had his growth spurt, and with puberty he wouldn't have to worry anymore. Was he supposed to be worrying now?

Ivy let him know that while he might get tall and thin, he might not; but either way there was nothing to worry about. Although girls received more messages about beauty and sexuality, Ivy noticed that her boy got plenty about attractiveness and athleticism. While eating disorders are still more prevalent in females, males are catching up, and Ivy was well aware that an important part of her job as a mother was to make sure her son didn't develop one—as she had and as had nearly everyone in her family.

He didn't, and Ivy would have known because she is an expert, both personally and professionally. She kept an eye out for whether he was sneaking, binge eating, or using food in ways that seemed to be overcompensating or self-soothing. But his relationship with food remained perfectly healthy. He stopped eating when he was full. He could say no to desserts when he wasn't in the mood. He could eat one cookie, and not the whole bag. Still he was chubby, just as she had been. Ivy realized that if she had been left alone to be the chubby kid she was, she would not have developed an eating disorder or started weight cycling—dieting and then overeating when she wasn't dieting, and then dieting again. Frankly, raising her son was an experiment in parenting, the first generation of learning from a family's mistakes. And the mistakes her family made had not only been significant, but public.

Nearly everyone in Ivy's family was big. Her sisters, her parents, her aunts, and her cousins. In fact, her first cousin was professionally big—she was "Big Mama Cass." They were a family genetically prone to being big, and much to their disconcertion that perceived flaw was known to an international audience.

Ivy first came to understand that she was big in the fourth grade. Up until that point, she had no idea anything was awry. She knew that her mother hated her own body, because she was forever dieting. But mothers in the 1960s were all taking diet pills, and hers was no exception. Though up until Ivy was nine, she thought disdain for one's body was solely an adult concern. However, she learned from several sources that, in fact, little girls should begin to hate themselves at a young age. First, a family friend teased her: You have big legs, legs like a man. Like a man? There was clearly something terribly wrong. And then her cousin's success became a warning to them all. If Ivy wasn't careful, she was told, she would end up just like cousin Cass. Not famous. Not talented. Not wealthy. Not living in Beverly Hills. But, fat. Horribly, shamefully, fat.

Is it needless to say that this made little sense to a nine-year-old? Cass was a star. She was in the Mamas and the Papas now. She was arguably the best singer in the group. She was a close personal friend to Crosby, Stills and Nash, and the Monkees. Ivy adored the Monkees. Her older cousin was, to her, and to so many others, a superstar. What could possibly be wrong with someone like that? But from the family's perspective, Ellen Naomi Cohen, or "Mama Cass Elliot," was a fat girl, and worse yet, a fat girl that everyone could, and should, judge. Her success was completely eclipsed by her body. All else was erased. She would only truly be successful if she were thin. She was not like the Partridge Family girls, or her contemporaries in *Seventeen* magazine, and she certainly wasn't like her willowy band mate Michelle Phillips. Everybody wanted to be like Michelle Phillips.

Ivy is the youngest of three sisters. The eldest was always very fat and the middle sister was overweight but constantly, and is to this day, testing one more drastic diet. She gets plastic surgery and does everything possible to sculpt her body into something acceptable. That may or may not rival the eldest, who took the lap-band surgery plunge at age 60. It didn't help. In retrospect, Ivy realizes that she spent a great deal of her childhood and adolescent years not doing things she wanted to, because she felt she was too fat to do them.

Being pregnant was the first time in her life she believed she was sanctioned to be a fat person. It was the first time since she was a small child that she donned a bathing suit. As she was enveloped by the freedom of the water, she swam, and as she swam, so did her son, inside the safety of her womb. She vowed at that moment he would never miss the adventures that were lost to her because of shame. He would not be a victim of her self-hate. That meant she had to sanction him to love his body, no matter what its size. It also meant that she had to be willing to join him on adventures, no matter what her size.

As is so often the case, when Ivy looks back at pictures of herself as a child—in the fourth grade when she first learned she was fat—she wasn't in actuality fat at all. Athletic, stocky, muscular, husky. With red hair and freckles. Not a girl's girl, but a tomboy. When she hit adolescence, she became rounder. She grew large breasts and hips. Her butt was big, like every butt in her family. Tiny waist, curvy thighs. She wasn't thin, she wasn't a grown version of a tomboy, she was a woman. Instead of that, though, she was told she was fat. Her job now, as she understood it, was to somehow genetically mutate—grow six inches, lengthen her legs, slender her arms, compact her hips. Of course that never happened, but she did manage to develop a powerful hatred for that which she couldn't change. She succeeded at personal disappointment and disgust.

Ivy's cousin Cass was about ten years older than Ivy. Her burden, though passed down as efficiently as possible, was far worse. Of course she was critiqued by the public, but she was condemned by the family. She also became the role model for all things done wrong. "You don't want to eat that dessert; you'll end up like Cass." She was the bogeyman of all things body. And like any bogeyman, she was hideous. Ivy hadn't yet matured and failed to see how a fat body made her ugly. And worse, undesirable. Or even more tragic, a failure. Weren't there any fat successes? At ten, all Ivy could conceive of was Santa Claus. Every teen magazine article would mention Cass's weight, and even more humiliating, compare her to Michelle. There was gossip and innuendo, love triangles with Cass on the outside looking in, judgment from those she loved. It was all documented for posterity. And the world knew. Ivy knew it from a different perspective, though, from her cousin and friend, in an intimate way that tattlers don't portray. Cass's feelings were exactly what one would imagine they would be, her insecurities and disappointments those of an actual person. Too private for a loving cousin and family member in arms to exploit, but obvious enough even without the details.

The tragic irony of cousin Cass, or in retrospect, one of the tragic ironies, was that her family was not so much proud of her success, but more accurately, amazed. It must have been a fluke, and if she cared to savor it for any time, she had better change. That of course is another irony about Cass Elliot: to maintain what she had received, she had to change. Her own family didn't take her seriously; they were dismissive, because they were just like her. Aunt Bessie, Cass's mother, was a fat woman, too, and she didn't have success. Her older sister was a fat woman, and she didn't have success. Clearly, in their eyes, they were all the same.

And frankly, the world supported this. Every time Cass lost weight it was news. And she did lose weight, over and over. In fact she had lost weight before she died, and that was news. But not as much news as how she died. The story is well known: She was first said to have choked on a ham sandwich. Whatever the source, that was an additional irony about Big Mama Cass. It turned out not to be true. The official cause of death was a heart attack from being fat: "fatty myocardial degeneration due to obesity." And this is another irony about Cass Elliot. The public was aware that Cass had used drugs, including heroin. She had admitted as much. The reason for the drug use was not made so clear.

After all, drug use by musicians is not exactly unheard of. But heroin for weight loss was not so much discussed, and Cass didn't send out a press release. Some in her family knew better, and at her death, she had a small child whom they wished to protect. No one who cares wants a little girl to have a mother who died of an overdose. There is no proof, but Ivy knows. Many have tried to spin her death. It has been claimed that her heart was weakened from dieting, or officially, she literally died from fat. And she did, but the delivery system was not a ham sandwich, or many ham sandwiches, and it wasn't exactly dieting, in a typical sense. But it was from an effort to lose weight, in the way she did it best, like a rock star.

Ivy was put on her first formal diet in junior high school; she was sent to Weight Watchers. She was five feet tall and weighed about 125 pounds. Her family thought she was very fat, but at least she looked like them. Tragically her mother died when Ivy was thirteen and her father married a woman even more zealous about weight. She also looked very different from Ivy, and was the antithesis of Ivy's mom. She was lean and weighed herself daily. If she gained a single pound she would fanatically diet for two days. Ivy's new role model was not only sharply focused on fat but was also an entirely different physical archetype. That's when Ivy began using diet pills. These were prescription pills from a doctor, and they were very effective, if the goal was getting a whole lot done, fast. Her schoolwork improved, or at least got finished faster, and she did lose weight. But when the weight came off she figured she was fixed—people finally thought she was pretty and she got heaps of attention. Goal met. She stopped the pills and as quickly as the weight came off, it came back on, plus more. Of course.

Even so, Ivy wasn't all that fat, but there didn't seem to be grades of fat back then, other than pass-fail. No one was a little fat, there was no chubby for girls. You were all right, or you were fat. So Ivy was fat. Ivy's best friend was 30 pounds heavier than she was, but there was no sense of envy for Ivy. There were no degrees. Her friend was fat, Ivy was fat, they were both fat. How fat didn't matter. And really, there were pragmatic reasons for this. If you couldn't buy your clothing in the regular store, if you couldn't wear the fashions of the day; if your blue jeans were purchased from a special place, it wasn't particularly relevant what size you bought at the fat-girl shop.

It didn't help that her father was fat, too. He was also a constant dieter. Dieting wasn't just for the women. He went on Atkins and Pritikin's, the grapefruit diet, any fad, and he encouraged everyone to join him. By encouraged, that is, he led his daughters to believe that the only measure of success for them was the size of their bodies, which he still does today, when the girls are more than a little grown. A great deal of damage was done. No one ever managed to keep the weight off. Ivy's sister, the one who failed at the lap band at 60, recently announced she has joined Weight Watchers, again. At 65. She needs knee surgery, and the doctors won't perform it on such a fat woman. Apparently, if you're fat and a failure, no matter how many ways you have tried, you made your own bed and should not be given the opportunity to walk to it.

Eating disorders were a family affair as well, or so it seemed. Everybody had one. It might not have been labeled as such at the time, but all the sisters and their father exhibited classic binge eating disorder behaviors, or what might have been called compulsive overeating, not to mention some other related issues that are not discussed in polite company. This led to a very interesting question for Ivy: Clearly there was a genetic component to weight, but was there also a genetic component to binge eating? Many people consider compulsive eating to be an addiction. In fact, Overeaters Anonymous bases its entire model on this notion.

As a therapist, Ivy notes that there are three components to addiction and substance abuse: a genetic predisposition, local environmental influence, and a larger societal impact. Five people could have a drink, but it is the person who is genetically predisposed to alcoholism, has family members who drink excessively, and lives where drinking is sanctioned by the community who is most likely to develop alcoholism. This may be a simplification, but it serves as a useful comparison. If a person is genetically predisposed to being fat, ridiculed, and forced to go on diets, while living in an environment filled with excess (not only of food but of weight-loss programs), perhaps food becomes a substance like alcohol. Is the brain chemistry involved in addiction to alcohol the same as that which makes ice cream self-soothing? Probably not, so addiction to food is not precisely the same as addiction to alcohol, and alcoholism is not precisely akin to binge eating disorder—but it certainly is an interesting comparison with some logical merit. Additionally, it is not uncommon for someone who has had weight-loss surgery, and can no longer consume certain foods, to develop other substance issues. On the other hand, few might care about binge eating itself if it didn't lead to fatness. Certainly Ivy's family wouldn't have. The food wasn't inherently bad, but the fat was horrendous.

Eventually Ivy did recover from her eating disorder, though the process was intensive. It required, among other very difficult endeavors, that she stop hating her body. She called a truce. She stopped dieting. She also acknowledged what comfort food did for her, and that to need comfort is not contemptible, but natural. She says that eating is a way to be nurtured from the inside, and there is nothing wrong with that. The problem lies with the guilt a person feels after they eat the ice cream because they are lonely, and when it's gone they are still lonely. Many stop there, with the logic that ice cream does not solve loneliness. That is not the true key, however. It is not that eating ice cream and still feeling lonely is an offense. Eating ice cream may not cure loneliness, but it is still nurturing from the inside. The true dilemma is that guilt causes shame, and shame makes us feel not only lonely, but unlovable. The feeling of being unlovable is the true culprit, the catalyst in the cycle, and why Ivy made it her mission to prevent her son from experiencing the intolerable sense of being unlovable.

The primary way Ivy made sure her son felt lovable was to make sure he felt loved, and to make sure he loved others. She says her son was born into an environment of self-acceptance with no apology. He was surrounded by every kind of person, of every size, shape, color, and orientation. For him, to be normal was to be different. When he was teased in school for being fat he felt more curiosity than pain. How strange to revile a person for the way they looked. How sad for the person who didn't know better. No one likes to be mocked, but one's own reaction has most of the power. Ivy's son was teased, but he was not obliterated by the attack. He was called gay, too, and though not gay, he loved people who were. Ivy says:

> I'll never forget when he came home from school and said, "It's not that I mind that they're calling me gay; what bothers me is they think it's an insult." And I think that's how he felt about fat, too. He said, "They can call me what they want, but it's really horrible that they think fat is an insult, that's what's wrong, that we think that fat and gay is an insult, or white or black is an insult, that's where the problem is, not the fact that I'm fat," which to this day makes me cry.

As any proud mama would.

2

IF I WERE A HAT I WOULD BE A SOMBRERO

Though it hadn't been in her life plan, Elaine became a stepmother to four children, all under ten years of age. This was not a mission for the faint of heart. Even under the best of circumstances, four little kids from parents who have split are bound to have some unresolved issues. These little kids were no exception.

Elaine became part of the family at record speed. By their second date, the father of these children determined they should all convene, and he arranged a family outing. Of course Elaine was anxious, but this meet-and-greet proved trickier than she had even imagined. In the stands of the baseball game where they sat, the baby of the family, three years old, crawled into her lap and promptly asked Elaine if she would be his mommy. The next in line, a girl age five, also snuggled up close. The older daughter, age seven, on the other hand, wanted nothing to do with Elaine and was pleased to have her daddy all to herself. And the eldest, Paul, eight years old, didn't care much about her, or his dad, or the game. He just wanted a snack.

Though tempting, Elaine tried not to draw any specific conclusions. Two needy young ones, a daddy's girl, and a husky older brother could mean something, or it could mean nothing at all.

A short time later, it was Christmastime, and Elaine was expected at the festivities. Of course she came bearing gifts. But it was nothing fancy, just some baby-sized socks on which she embroidered their names—then she filled them with trinkets. For each a toy car, a bouncy ball, and some hard candy. Not the kind of loot one might expect from Santa himself, but a thoughtful gift, nonetheless. As it turned out, Elaine outdid Santa by a mile. Not only did the kids covet these dime-store toys, but the youngest collected all the socks and wore them, as socks. It became difficult for Elaine not to start being suspicious.

When she first met Paul, the eldest, he was larger than average boys, though she didn't think much of it. There were plenty of boys his age and his size. However, it quickly became apparent that Paul exhibited some behaviors that weren't so average. For one, he seemed to be unaware of when he had eaten; literally, he couldn't recall. He also claimed to always be hungry, and he anxiously anticipated every next meal. If the family would go for a buffet dinner, during which he had eaten copious amounts of food, on the drive home, with all innocence, he would ask if they could stop for burgers. He seemed to honestly forget he had just eaten. To add to that, Paul would eat large quantities of whatever food happened to be available.

In short order, Paul grew to 140 pounds. At only nine years old, he was heavier than Elaine. Within the next few years, Paul tripled his body size, and by the time he was a teenager, he weighed approximately 450 pounds.

They never knew exactly how much Paul weighed because none of the medical scales, not even those of the bariatric doctor, could record his actual weight. Paul was sent to specialists, anyone who would see him. Elaine assumed he must have some kind of medical condition, and so did all of the medical professionals. At each visit, the doctor would proclaim to know exactly what was wrong with Paul—he must be diabetic, or have a hormonal disorder, or perhaps a genetic condition. But when the tests returned, it turned out doctor after doctor was wrong. Physically, apart from his size, Paul was completely normal.

Since there appeared to be nothing medically wrong with Paul, and obesity did not run in the family, everyone assumed it must be psychological. But why? And it's not like Paul was a couch potato. He was in fact quite an active kid. He played outside with his brother and sisters, he ran around just as much as the others. He took karate, as they all did, and could perform a side high kick above his head. He was athletic. In fact so athletic, that combined with his size, he was not permitted to spar with children his own age. He was put in a karate class with adults, grown men with beards, and although he was perfectly skilled for his age, and even larger than most of the men, he was still just a boy. The experience was intimidating and even sometimes frightening.

Nevertheless, Paul liked to be macho. Paul enjoyed shooting BB guns, and he even learned to use a crossbow. When visiting his grandfather's ranch, he was in his element. Paul was a boy's boy, and he didn't seem to mind that his size aided in that impression.

In fact, it was evident that Paul used his size as self-protection, and to protect his brother and sisters. His mother's neighborhood was different from his father's. It was tough and the kids were subjected to the whims of bullies. At five years old, one of his sisters was attacked by a group of seven-year-old street toughs. They were just children, but had it not been for Paul pulling them off her, and scaring the ever-loving daylights out of them, she could have been seriously hurt. That was not the only time he used his size to his advantage. At one point or another, each of his siblings needed rescuing. Paul was an intimidating figure with his physical presence and dominating character. Being big, in size and disposition, were characteristics Paul seemed to covet, and it appeared, at least, that he worked both consciously and subconsciously to obtain his stature and maintain it.

It is impossible to say whether the need to become extra-large was initially an unconscious drive or a rational decision, but it clearly was important to him. In middle school Paul gained weight quickly, dramatically, and apparently intentionally. It seemed from the way he spoke about hunger that Paul did not have a reliable internal sensor for fullness, though he also actively worked at gaining weight. More than once, Elaine found Paul with half of a sandwich in his hand while simultaneously complaining that he hadn't eaten anything all day. When it was pointed out that he was holding partially eaten food, he was genuinely surprised. It was as if he immediately forgot he had eaten each time he ate. While it was not clear if Paul registered it even as he was eating, he had an uncanny ability to remember all the food from his past. He would reminisce with acute detail about some sandwich he ate in Florida a year ago, while forgetting the one eaten a minute before.

This was not an intellectual deficit. Paul was very bright; he was in advanced classes in all his subjects. It also wasn't a con. As long as no one was overtly trying to make him lose weight, he didn't hide his eating. It seemed more as if he had some kind of emotional block, though for a long time there was no explanation for it.

The situation was even worse when Paul was at his mother's— plus there was less supervision there. During that time he was often truant. Paul would go to school, but immediately come home and climb into his house through the window, while his mother was at work. He would then proceed to eat literally whatever was available to be eaten. He would eat whole loaves of bread and entire sticks of butter. A compulsion of some kind? Possibly, but not entirely. It was also a mission. Paul needed to be large, and then larger.

There were times when Elaine's husband would be away and she would have Paul to herself for a period of weeks. Elaine would attempt armchair behavior modification. Her favorite tactic was to delay. She would hold off on snack time for fifteen minutes, then suggest that it was too close to dinner for a snack. Elaine would also monitor his food, though in a way that Paul did not seem to notice, or at least not mind. She would prepare food, giving Paul limited choices—a snack might be either an apple or some cottage cheese. They would sit down together and eat, and if he wanted more, she would say sure, and offer him a little bit of whatever she felt most healthful. It wasn't a diet exactly and there was no discussion of weight loss. It was an attempt at moderation, which, frankly, nobody likes and almost anyone would notice and resent. Interestingly, Paul did not seem to have any problem with it. He didn't complain or act deprived. He was perfectly cheerful about the entire thinly veiled process.

That is, until his father mentioned that Paul seemed to have dropped a few pounds. This would send him into a panic. At the mere mention that Paul appeared smaller, he would head directly to the kitchen and consume everything and anything that he could find. This would recur if anyone, at any point, stated that Paul looked slimmer, more toned, or "good" in any way. The notion that he had dropped the slightest amount of weight was a catalyst for remedying the situation as quickly and efficiently as possible. Again, it wasn't obvious whether Paul was acting on instinct or making a conscious decision. But it was crystal clear that Paul had no intention of becoming smaller than his approximately 450 pounds—which seemed to be the magic number, the one that was just above what registered on the scale.

Paul was not a closet eater, as he made no attempt to hide his bingeing or constant longing for more to eat—that is, until he was put on a diet. On a formal regime prescribed by a doctor, Paul became someone who sneaked food. Elaine would find evidence of this when she changed his sheets—unearthing a graveyard of Popsicle sticks and melted ice cream that was buried under the mattress. Doctors had no idea what to do with Paul. There was no potion or pill, and diets were a total bust. Whether or not Paul felt any internal conflict about being so large was not evident. He didn't seem to be embarrassed by his size. Although, Elaine was reasonably certain he was teased at school, and of course he was. They had to buy his clothing in a big and tall men's shop, which would fit him horizontally but vertically would hang past his fingers and toes. In his teens he took to wearing T-shirts when swimming, but it wasn't to cover girth. He had stretch marks so deep people would ask him about the injury that caused the scars. There was little Elaine could do to protect him from any of this. She ensured his siblings didn't tease him while at her house, but they didn't anyway, and that was about all she could do.

Although Paul was not harassed about his size when Elaine was present, she believes he was mocked somewhere. Most certainly at school and she suspects by his mother. By chance one time Elaine came upon a school assignment Paul left lying around. He and his classmates were asked to pick a hat style that most represented them, and explain why. Paul's paper stated, "If I were a hat I would be a sombrero, because I am big and lazy." Paul was big, but he wasn't lazy. Elaine tried to comfort him; she assured him that he wasn't lazy at all. Paul's retort was that he was stupid, too.

Paul was not stupid, he was quite sharp, and even more so, charming and funny. Paul was witty and good-spirited with an excellent sense of humor. He was an avid joke teller, memorizing and reciting the entire routines of his favorite comedians. Though he never made fat jokes. He never laughed at his own size—there was no self-deprecating humor. Being fat was, for some reason, serious business.

Whether or not there was a negative emotional impact on Paul because of his size, it did seem to impact his younger sisters. At five years old, one of the girls developed a fixation about having cellulite on her thighs. Both sisters regularly claimed they were dieting while still in elementary school. Though some of this behavior may have been influenced by the general cultural obsession with girls and thinness, they seemed to be particularly concerned. It was more pronounced, different. Not that the girls claimed their brother was a trigger—they didn't speak of his weight. But Elaine believed Paul was the source of their concern. Eventually, Elaine and their father got custody and she raised the girls full time. She helped them to stop obsessing about their weight, with good success.

It was during the battle for custody that many of the mysteries began to unravel, the secrets kept between the children and their mother, and why Paul was, well, the way he was. There had been telltale signs. Precursors to the big reveal. Oddities. For instance, Paul never had socks. He would come to visit Elaine and her husband, and each time, Paul would be missing his socks. It was a bone of contention because invariably they would purchase him a new jumbo pack replacement, and somehow the next time, they would be mislaid again. Paul couldn't, or wouldn't, say why. Paul's younger brother developed a peculiar habit of hand washing his own socks, and would sleep with them under his pillow. He was more forthcoming with an explanation. He matter-of-factly told Elaine he was protecting them, so his mother would not cut them up with scissors. Their mother had been systematically destroying all the socks to cause conflict during their father's visitation. Why the children had neglected to share this information was not yet clear.

There were other issues as well. The children never seemed to have clean or intact clothing, in general. During one visit, Paul showed up with only the shirt on his back, a ripped tee covered in tire tracks. Tire tracks. It's not like Elaine's husband was a deadbeat dad. He paid child support, but mysteriously, somehow, the money was not getting to the kids. They had nothing. Their mother, on the other hand, was always sharp as a tack, with coiffed hair, and accessorized. The little girls' hair never seemed to be brushed, which made them terribly self-conscious, and Elaine would spend hours getting the knots out. They became anxious about perfection, and not surprisingly so, because when they went to school from their mother's house, they were completely disheveled, and teased mercilessly. All the kids frequently had lice or fleas, which their mother tried to rid with dog shampoo. It was traumatic to be told they were not worthy of having a shampoo for humans. The youngest boy, so disturbed by the idea, became terrified of water altogether. It took months for Elaine to convince him to let her wash his hair in the sink.

Altogether, their mother's home was a disaster. There were never any clean dishes, so the kids took to eating directly off the carpet. Each time Elaine and her husband would pick up the children for a visit, they complained of being starving, so they would show up with bags and bags of fast-food, which the children would proceed to dump right on the rug, their regular eating surface. Also, these kids would eat anything put in front of their hungry faces. They were certainly not raised as foodies, and it was always a surprise to Elaine when a first grader would gladly devour something like blue cheese.

Clearly these children were neglected, but it wasn't until one Christmas visit that it was finally revealed they were also abused. Simply put, their mother beat them. Elaine was busy putting together a do-it-yourself picture frame for the holiday and the younger boy, seeing the wood with points on either end, said, in his innocent "that's life" sort of fashion, "That's just like Mom's spanking stick." Their mother had been abused herself, and perhaps in a feeble attempt to justify continuing the pattern, she portrayed her experiences as a badge of honor. "You have no right to complain; it was much worse for me." Elaine and their father did not send the children back after that Christmas visit, and so began the battle for custody.

Elaine and her husband hired a lawyer and filed for custody. There was a court hearing in which Paul was required to testify against his mother—he was eleven years old, and terrified. Despite his testimony and myriad other pieces of evidence, the judge determined that "every mother should get a second chance," and he ordered the children be returned to her. At that ruling, this scene followed: The youngest, a five-year-old girl, shot like a bat out of hell from the courthouse into downtown traffic, with her father frantically following to prevent her from getting hit by a car. Simultaneously, the next oldest, a boy, managed to hide by squirming into a tiny space behind the vending machine in the lobby, where no adult-size person could reach him. The older girl grabbed Elaine by the torso and legs and clung to her for dear life; all the while friends of the mother were yelling at Elaine about kidnapping and such dramatic nonsense. Elaine stretched her arms up in the air to demonstrate she had no force on the child, but the girl remained latched on. And Paul, he just slunk to the floor. He appeared to be in some kind of stupor, perhaps in shock. He was motionless, silent, and devastated. Their father's lawyer, in a highly unorthodox move, pleaded with the judge as this drama unfolded. It was mayhem. But custody was decided. At least the judge had also assured there were to be regular visits from child protective services and mandatory family counseling. Small favors.

As it turned out, the intervention of the social worker was far more than a small favor. Family counseling was highly productive, and shortly thereafter, the counselor managed to convince the mother to give up custody. The tactics are unknown. So all of the children packed up their rags and went to live with their father and Elaine. Though it took time, the children seemed to recover, each of them, except for Paul. He had spent nine years alone with his mother, enough time for abuse to scar. He continued to weigh around 450 pounds, though he seemed to stabilize at that weight. Just heavy enough not to register on the scales, clearly signifying something, but no one was sure what.

However, with the custody battle and the truth about the abuse, it finally emerged why Paul needed to be the size that he was, and he did indeed need to be that size. He had never intended to reveal his motivation; in fact it's not even clear how conscious that motivation was to him. But those around him drew a conclusion, one that, frankly, had become profoundly and extraordinarily obvious. Whether Paul would acknowledge this as truth, we will never know.

Paul's mother would rage, wielding her spanking stick and other tools of destruction. The children would run, hiding in any room they could escape to before getting attacked. But there was only so much protection the floor under a bed or clothes hanging in a closet could offer. This is where Paul came in. At 450 pounds, at precisely this weight, Paul was the perfect size to fill a doorway. He became a living wall, an immovable barrier, to prevent their abusive mother from reaching the children tucked away in an otherwise defenseless pose. He took the wrath upon himself in a grand posture to save the small ones who had no defense. He was their bodyguard. He guarded their bodies with his own. Malleable but the perfect size for the job, he filled any space, molded when necessary, but was always solid. Flesh and bone and muscle, he was an impenetrable gate. Whether consciously or not, Paul had built the perfect tool for the job. The perfect size, the perfect fit, the perfect structure.

If Paul was a hat he wasn't a sombrero. He was a hood, with a mask and cape, because Paul was a superhero, and his special power was being fat. Also, like so many superheroes, no one was aware of his dual identity. In this case, not even he.

By the time Paul was a junior in high school Elaine and her husband had split. The counselor told Elaine that the children had already been abandoned too many times and she advised Elaine not to initiate contact. Most likely, terrible advice. Nonetheless Elaine heeded her recommendation. Elaine didn't hear from any of them for decades. It's not that they didn't love her or miss her, but expecting broken children to instigate a long-distance relationship, well, the obvious occurred. Eventually, though, the children grew up and the youngest girl sent Elaine an email. The kids felt guilty for not being more appreciative and Elaine felt guilty for leaving them as she did. It was a touching and happy ending as they keep in regular contact, all the children, step-grandchildren, and Elaine. Except for Paul.

The three younger kids, now adults with families of their own, are all close. They live nearby each other, provide mutual love and support, form a bonded community, and none are in contact with Paul. They have tried; he isn't interested. They don't speak to their father or mother, either, which is not terribly surprising. But through some family grapevine they have heard that Paul is still weighing in at 450 pounds and lives in his maternal childhood home, with his mother. No one knows if he ever had any outside relationships or a family of his own. Or more important, why a superhero would return to the scene of the crime. Perhaps he still mistakes his hood, mask, and cape for a sombrero.

3

FAT IMMUNITY

The "President's Physical Fitness Test" has been the bane of every fat kid's existence since President Lyndon B. Johnson introduced it in 1966. Addison remembers vividly the moment she became conscious of being fat. It was the third grade and her first experience with the president's test. For a couple of weeks, all the kids were tested: How many pull-ups can you do? How fast can you run a mile? How long can you jump rope? The particular exercises are of no consequence really. What made it so memorable for Addison was the public competition—how she compared seemed to reflect her inherent goodness as a child. And then there is the weigh-in.

Addison was the heaviest person in the school. At eight or nine years old, she was 95 pounds. She knew it, and all the other kids knew it, because the weighing took place in front of everyone. Not even a shame curtain separated her from her gawking peers. And needless to say, the heaviest kid in the school, a fat girl, heard no end. She was made fun of, of course. She was terribly embarrassed, of course. She felt very fat for the first time in her life, and painfully conscious of her body, of course. And of course, that was just the beginning.

Prior to that incident, the children hadn't fully comprehended the power of teasing; it was as if by realizing Addison was fat and telling her so struck a chord, they had a glorious awakening. They learned the intense authority of being cruel. Before that, they rather pitifully made fun of each other for a lackluster array of Pokémon cards or an obsolete Barbie. No one had yet realized that jabs regarding another person's body were potent, satisfying, and for the majority of them, who were inconspicuously average, made them immune.

Of course, the irony that the president's test was supposed to support children in using and feeling good about their bodies—and instead Addison became desperate to hide hers in shame—wasn't lost on even an eight-year-old. It was, however, apparently lost on the adults, because Addison's indignity was thirty years after they implemented the thing—several generations of institutionalized humiliation later.

Like a bolt of lightning on a clear day, a new playground discussion sparked. Previously, the most biting of insults might regard smelly gym socks or outdated fashion choices. But there had never been a hierarchy of bodies before. They had never before discussed each other's size and shape, much less the number of pounds associated with it. With the introduction of that scale, the children were given an entirely new tool to rationalize good and bad, and they seemed to have in innate ability to capitalize on it. It was the first day of the rest of Addison's life. Never again would she be just a kid. Now she was a fat kid. And that's an entirely different life experience.

Besides the results of the weigh-in being her initiation to being labeled "overweight," it was the first time Addison was exposed to any consciousness about fitness. Now, that's largely the intent of the program. Sadly, fitness seemed to have a pass-fail grading system, which was not particularly conducive to working toward gradual improvement. No one ever introduced the idea of "healthy" as being related to actual health, or that it might be on a continuum. It is true that one could improve at exercise, or lose weight over time, but there was a line in the sand that indicated good versus bad. The President's Physical Fitness Test had winners and losers. It still does today. This was particularly shocking to Addison, because weight and fitness had never been an issue in her home. Not because everyone was slim and in fine form, but because no one was, and no one cared. There was no weight consciousness in Addison's home, so it never before occurred to her that she was deficient.

Both of Addison's parents had weight "issues." Her father has always been extremely large. Her mother has yo-yoed throughout her life. She's not so much a dieter, but is very prone to emotional weight cycling. When in poor spirits, she would lose weight. But when things were going well and she catered to her husband's big appetite, she would gain weight keeping up. There also wasn't any particular concern for the kinds of foods they ate, other than it should taste good. There was virtually no home cooking. Pizza and fast food were staples. A common meal was procured when her father would use the drive-through at McDonald's and buy two dozen cheeseburgers, then dole them out in the car as he saw fit at that moment. Addison might get one, or three. She grabbed candy bars if she was hungry. It was a bad cliché of the American diet, and really, no one would argue it was a healthful way to live, or raise a child.

As far as Addison can tell, her weight was a combination of factors that brewed the perfect storm: genetic predisposition, no understanding of nutrition or portion control, and emotional eating, which she witnessed in her parents and seemed inherently logical—eating felt good. It wasn't long before Addison developed an eating disorder. In her entire life, Addison has no memory of not being big, and doesn't expect to ever experience skinny.

There were other factors, particular to Addison's life. She has three siblings, but they are much older, so Addison was essentially raised as an only child. Her father was agoraphobic and rarely went outside. Then because of the AMBER Alert frenzy during her childhood, she wasn't allowed out much either. When she became old enough to drive, she secured a certain amount of freedom, but by then the die had been cast. There hadn't been much opportunity to play with other children in her youth, so she didn't exactly develop into a social butterfly busting from her cocoon.

For better or worse, the adults most directly in her life were matter-of-fact about her weight and the ritual of being weighed. At school the process was regimented: Kids lined up, weighing occurred, the number was announced then scribbled in a chart, and the child was sent off to jump rope. If teachers or nurses or other grown-ups were concerned about Addison's weight, they didn't show it. The blasé attitude of the adults didn't stop the children from latching tightly onto the numbers when they were read off the scales. And it didn't stop the schoolyard scandal. But there was not yet an obsession with making those fat kids thin. Of course, there are differences between wanting to make someone thin and judging her because she is fat, especially if you don't actually know her.

The teachers and school nursing staff didn't have to take ownership of the fat kids back then, because they weren't being blamed, yet. But parents were encouraged to accept that their child's appearance was a direct reflection of themselves. This is why Addison believes the kids cared so much about the numbers—it was their reaction to life in a continual beautiful baby competition. Dieting mothers and advertisers had long since picked up on weight loss as a cash cow. So while those close to her were pretty much silent, the gawkers from afar had a thing or two to say.

> I've thought about it a lot over the years. I think maybe there was a cultural perspective that most of those kids were raised with that I wasn't. I wasn't raised in a household where weight was something to be conscious of, where people were constantly evaluated by how skinny or fat they were, where it was a positive or negative thing to be looked at or analyzed. So I feel like the children picked up that attitude somewhere I wasn't. Maybe they did grow up in houses where people were actively dieting or constantly watching their weight and eating vegetables. Maybe it's something they picked up from TV, where all

of the heroines were skinny and beautiful and all of the villains were fat and balding. That was never in my head. My reaction was pure shame.

Addison felt she was branded by these scandalous numbers, and she was. Her way of coping was to bully those even weaker than herself.

Any child in that situation would want to escape that however they could. I escaped it, honestly, by making fun of the people who weighed more than me. If there was a kid who had a reputation for being mean or was made fun of for other reasons then I would join in on that. I would try to make sure it was clear which side of that line I was on. If I couldn't be skinny at least I could pick the stronger side. It was a kill or be killed mentality. I tried to stay neutral, I never aligned myself with any cliques or groups, but if it ever came to scapegoating anyone else, I would engage in it.

Since that fateful day in gym class, weight was perpetually in Addison's consciousness and her subconscious. And then came puberty. She hit puberty early, the next year. By the fourth grade, she had reached her maximum height of five foot three and developed all there was to develop. She was about a foot and a half taller than her peers, which meant that even without "extra" weight she weighed considerably more than her classmates, though for Addison there was also "extra" weight involved. She wore size 13 pants and had a wide frame. She was large for a ten-year-old girl, no matter how you sliced it.

That worked well for her in one aspect of life. Addison was a soccer player and feared by her competitors. They expected her to bulldoze them down. It was a double-edged sword. She was always stuck in the back as a defender. She couldn't run very fast and huffed and puffed when she did, but as the defense she was a powerhouse. The other girls didn't want to get anywhere close to her, and if she was near the goal, the other team was far away from it. She got a certain amount of positive reinforcement for this, but it was, through no intention of her own, as a bully. "Addison, they whispered, 'she could beat you up.' I even got a little of that from my dad. My sheer size made me capable of doing a number on someone, if I wanted to." She was a badass, at least that is how it was presented to her. The terminator, respected for her power, at least the power they perceived she had.

Though that wasn't a persona she chose, she enjoyed it. It seemed positive, if only for the fact that people weren't making fun of her. She was no longer on the bottom rung of the social ladder. She had a status. She wasn't popular, rich, or pretty—she was that quietly intimidating kid. Intimidating being the operative word, and the only positive aspect she imagined she possessed. That lasted until the sixth or seventh grade, when her physical stature became far less impressive, relatively speaking.

At that point, Addison was forced to develop her personality. She was smart and got good grades. She rarely spoke, but when she did, she had the right answer. She found a new way to be intimidating: She took on a mysterious and standoffish demeanor. That wasn't entirely planned either, but she recognized it in herself. She knew that if she did not present vulnerabilities to exploit, they could not use them against her. Addison was reserved in what she said and did, giving everything forethought. Her mantra: Never look stupid. It worked—people viewed her as confident and even intimidating, though she didn't realize it, because it was all just a calculated effort not to be embarrassed as the fat girl. It was effective compensation, though more performance than reality. In her own mind, being careful and reserved was merely armor, not a weapon.

As for home life, not much changed. Her relationship with her mother was, has been, and still is, strong. Not so much with her father, with whom she butted heads. Her mother's attitude was always to accept Addison as she was. There was no pressure, overt or subtle, to change, and therein lies the fundamental reason they got along—unconditional love. Her father, though, who was much fatter than either Addison or her mother, did project some of his own dissatisfaction onto his daughter. Her childhood memories of him consisted nearly entirely of him planted on the couch, eating something. He was thin when he married Addison's mother, but his tendency to put on pounds, and her tendency to love people without judgment, resulted in considerable weight gain—at least that is a partial explanation.

Addison's parents met after her father's first divorce and radical self-created diet. Addison once found his secret recipe. He ate nothing but a soup made from chicken broth and celery. Needless to say, he dropped weight, and put it back on. It's not that Addison's father was explicitly critical of her. But she knew he saw himself in the girl—at least that is what she thinks she knows. He had been far more critical of Addison's older sister, who was also heavier than Addison. He bribed her with money for every pound she lost and then a follow-up shopping spree at the mall. This is a common, if not a clichéd, way to motivate youngsters to lose weight. It is always effective, for a few days, and later breeds contempt. He didn't use those tactics with Addison, but there were subtle cues. For instance, when he would buy those bags of cheeseburgers, how many Addison was given was a direct result of his feelings about her weight at the time. He also called her "Bubble Butt," which he claims was meant to aggravate Addison in a loving fatherly sort of way—although in retrospect, she wonders.

Addison didn't actively diet as a child. She didn't feel like "there was a skinny person inside her waiting to come out." Whatever ridicule she received, it seemed to be for something that could not be changed any more so than her eye color. She has always imagined herself as fat—that is simply who she is. She has felt guilt about it, and shame, but never the ability to change it. In high school, there was some desperate dieting—blind attempts for acceptance. The pressure for a girl to look a certain way is at its peak. And, of course, she was at her most sensitive to outside opinion, as well as still ignorant about whether the criticism was right or wrong. Also, she stopped playing soccer, there were no more Girl Scouts, and any extracurricular social structure she had had disappeared. She developed the hermit persona.

Luckily, in high school there were places for "girls like her"— the marching band, theater tech, and the honor society. On the other side of the coin, though, even if she found a home for way-ward uncool kids, her self-consciousness was at an all-time high. Even nerds want to date, and more important, be considered dat-able. Others like her seemed to be having experiences, experi-ments, but Addison was not—a fact she was painfully aware of. No one appeared to be interested in her, at least no one made it known. She began to have a whole new sense of being unaccept-ed and unwanted—now she was rejected from love. It drove her, almost literally, crazy. And that insanity is what drove her to diet, or at least to attempt to diet.

With the plan of dieting formed in her head, Addison allowed herself thoughts of being beautiful and acceptable. Like them. She dreamed she would be sought after—a real girl. It was sophomore year when Addison first brought a Lean Cuisine to school in a bag lunch. And it was humiliating. She ate microwave broccoli that reeked from a paper box, while all the normal people ate chicken-fried steak and potatoes. But she did this for six months, and reached her lowest weight in years: 180 pounds. That weight suited her well. She was legitimately curvy. Still a bit chubby, but it worked for her. It was a tremendous struggle to get there, though. Addison was an emotional eater; she derived happiness from food, and to not have that outlet was difficult and confus-ing. Also, despite reaching her lowest weight, and despite looking good at it, it was only 8 pounds less than where she had begun. In six months of stringent dieting, she had lost 8 pounds. She had also entirely warped her perspective. She looked good with an 8-pound loss, but it was only 8 pounds. So what was the real problem? Her weight? Her perception? Her perception of weight?

She had no answers, but that was one of only two times in her life that Addison has dieted.

She could never figure out why she had lost only 8 pounds. She admits she had been eating high-sodium foods, and during Friday-night football games she allowed herself some of the free nachos awarded to the band at halftime. But, honestly, at all other times she maintained military strictness to her 1,200-calorie-a-day plan. She was active in marching band, which was no walk in the park—rather it was two to three hours of walking, five days a week, plus game performances and Saturday competitions. Addison could do nothing but chalk it up to all the muscle she was building, the processed diet foods, and in retrospect, a complete distortion of her body image to begin with. Perhaps she didn't even need to lose the 8 pounds she lost. But at the time, that was unfathomable.

After the diet crash and burn, Addison had a latent period, as she calls it. She was constantly morose about being lonely and unaccepted, that nobody wanted to be her boyfriend while everyone else had a boyfriend, and that she was generally miserably dejected. It didn't help that she was sixteen. She did whatever she could to stay busy: became the band treasurer, the head of the theater tech department, hunkered down in the National Honors Society, and even ran clothing drives for the poor. Then, the summer before her senior year, she went on what turned out to be the most romantic trip of her life—to the place in New Mexico where they did nuclear bomb testing. It was on that school field trip that she met her future husband (now ex).

He was the first and still only person who ever showed interest in Addison (though to be fair, they have just recently divorced). He was very ambitious about his pursuit of her and not the least bit coy. She was swept away with love, and the next thing she knew, she had dates and a boyfriend, and within a year a promise ring, which became an engagement ring, and then a wedding ring—all by the time Addison was twenty-one. His love was like a dream, exciting and very transformative. She used to joke that, "Before I met him, I was on track to be the strange hermit cat lady that frightened all the neighborhood kids, only with dogs.

And then came the metaphorical white horse." It derailed all her plans, in the best way.

When they met, Addison was at her lowest weight, the post-diet 180 pounds. "I wasn't skinny and by today's standards I'd be fat, but it was a flattering fat, if there is such a thing. And he loved me just that way." But Addison didn't stay a "flattering fat," at least not in her husband's eyes. Halfway through college her weight became an issue, and eventually, she says, it's what ended their marriage. But at the time, in high school, Addison was convinced that it was her boyfriend who had a problem—because he was attracted to her. "I had conditioned myself, or maybe I had been conditioned by the world I lived in, that I wasn't acceptable. I would aggravate him because he would say, 'You're beautiful,' and I would respond, 'No, I'm not.' I couldn't accept that he accepted me, and there he was accepting me for who I was and had always been. It didn't connect in my mind."

The perhaps ironic result of all that acceptance is Addison gained a tremendous amount of self-confidence, and with it a great deal of weight. When she went away to college, she was adored. That freed up her mental energy for emotional growth. She found she was making her way in the world and not being looked down upon. There was no criticism of her weight, and that led to Addison feeling independent and self-assured. She liked herself. By the time she had graduated college, she had put on 80 pounds, and didn't care. Her husband did. He was not at all happy with her weight gain. He asked her to lose it, to get skinny for him. To which Addison said, straight up, "No!" So he got himself a mistress.

Even more so than the mistress, Addison found his lack of unconditional love an affront. She found it shallow and petty. She asked him if it would be all right if she requested he start living at the gym, and get pumped and ripped, just because that's how she wanted him to look. He took offense to that. It was a vicious cycle. Soon after, he started a cyber affair, which turned into a plane ticket, which turned into the end of the marriage. Addison is only twenty-five now, so this was just a few short months ago.

Addison has moved back in with her parents. She is working to build herself up again. Much of that self-satisfaction she had built, when she felt loved, came tumbling down. Everything in shatters, Addison started dieting again—the second time in her life she has dieted. That dieting didn't last, as most diets don't. However, Addison has begun to examine her food choices in a new way. Even living at home, she no longer eats the way her parents raised her. Now it's organic and fresh food. She has lost about 60 pounds, which she calls a "side effect." Addison considers this a permanent lifestyle change, sees her life getting back on track. She wants to feel good "from the inside out. It's a symbolic cleansing."

Addison believes that she and her father are emotional eaters. "Food was a great way to smooth over a fight or polish over a perfect day. My memories of fun aren't complete without the pizza. And if I had a bad day, instead of taking a bubble bath, I would eat to feel better." Clearly, this is not unusual, and neither are attempts at "lifestyle changes." But Addison feels she is growing as a person, and that is exactly what every twenty-five-year-old should be trying to do.

Addison is truly not sure whether she wishes her parents raised her differently.

> On some levels, yes, I do wish my parents had done things differently. I wonder if my parents had instilled healthy eating habits in me, or encouraged me to go out and exercise, would I have been different? Would I have been prettier or healthier, would my marriage not have ended, would I have had other suitors? I wonder that, but I'm not mad at them for being anything other than what they were. And who knows what good things I would be losing, and what bad things I would gain, if things had been different? Maybe if they had instilled that as a kid, I would have worse body image and self-esteem issues than I already have—who knows?

I've always been an advocate that a person's body is not who they are. There is discrimination from all ends, but I have never believed that size should determine worth. I'd like to see our culture take a new turn; ever since I was a kid, I've seen the world turn to be more prejudiced and scathing toward the idea of fat, and to the people that fat is attached to. In my life I've seen so much hate and disgust and dismissiveness and people being treated as less than human. I'd like to see that change.

I'm not doing what I do now to lose weight. When I dieted, it was a punishment for being fat, a penance I had to pay in order to be absolved of the sin of fatness, and the way to find the enlightenment of being an acceptable size. I don't see the goal now as losing weight. I'm doing it because I want to be healthier and make better decisions. I started this when my life was spinning out of control. I could control what I ate; that was a way I could take hold of something. It wasn't punishment, it was a sense of control of my life.

And that's really all Addison can do, because physically and psychologically, there is no such fat immunity.

4

FLESHY AND BONES

Bettina's childhood nickname was Bones. She was unusually thin, worrisomely thin. Her mother would complain she didn't eat enough to keep a bird alive, and relatively speaking, this may well have been true. Then puberty hit. By sixth grade Bettina was one of maybe three girls who had breasts and hips. At the time, she felt like they might never stop growing, her womanly curves expanding from front to back and side to side.

It was around this time she noticed the fat boy in class. She, never having been fat herself, but now, if not fat, at least round, homed in on the one person more unusual than herself, and she was relentless. Though she didn't think of it as such at that time, Bettina was a bully. Part curious and part masochist, Bettina would ask the boy pointed questions about being fat, always going for the laugh, though certainly not from him. Bettina wasn't altogether bold in her display, but her ever-so-slightly shy delivery did not help to soften the blow. She was a more subtle bully, and as such, lashing back was a double-edged sword.

As Bettina was wont to do at that time, precocious and collecting material, she would read the dictionary for fun. Coming across the word *fleshy*, she assigned him that name for the entire school year, even from across the room. Though her somewhat awkward attempts at humiliation were more about drawing attention to herself, they were not without impact on Fleshy, the boy now identified as containing excess flesh.

Sadly ironic, Bettina wasn't exactly condemning Fleshy. She perceived her taunts as more like affectionate ribbing. Except she and Fleshy had not established affection for each other—they had never been friends. So what might have, though unlikely, been a bonding exercise was for Fleshy uncomfortable taunting. Even more ironic, and sad, in retrospect, Bettina realized that she probably had a crush on Fleshy and acts of bullying were some sort of misguided and misunderstood pigtail pulling, only much more painful, particularly coming from one of only a few girls with the power of their own flesh fully developed.

Decades later, Bettina has tried to find Fleshy, periodically searching through annual yearbooks and other reference material. She would like to speak with him, express that she is regretful. Perhaps that is born out of a selfish need for assurance that she did him no harm, and the revelation that the man he has likely become is now her romantic preference. Not to mention that Bettina herself has become quite fleshy; she is no longer Bones.

Though at his expense, Bettina's questions to Fleshy really did stem from some innate curiosity, at least in part. For instance, Bettina would see something in the news about food and weight and she would ask him what he eats. They weren't necessarily unkind at face value, but they were kids, not as able to recognize subtleties and interpretation, though many adults would be rightfully annoyed, and embarrassed, by the same kinds of questions—particularly when asked by someone who nicknamed you Fleshy. As far as interpretation goes, Bettina wasn't terribly sophisticated either. She didn't quite make the connection that there might be a social downside to being fat. She was curious about it. She didn't contemplate that he might suffer as a result of his size, that he might be ridiculed by others, that there were activities in which he could not participate. It wasn't until she was much older that Bettina realized she had been insensitive, naive, shortsighted, cruel, and a bully.

She wasn't lacking compassion; she honestly did not realize compassion was in order. As a twelve-year-old, she didn't fully realize she was making fun of him. As an adult, of course, she knows better. Upon reflection, Bettina realizes there are times and places where teasing is acceptable. Close family and friends with whom one shares a common bond, and knows each other's boundaries and sensitivities. But with a casual acquaintance, fewer liberties are taken, and in this case, Fleshy was a casual acquaintance at best, assuming twelve-year-olds even have casual acquaintanceships. In fact at twelve, Bettina didn't really have any kind of friendships with boys, not quite yet—and Fleshy, well, he didn't seem to have any friendships at all. So it is reasonable to suspect Bettina was neither the first nor the last to notice Fleshy's flesh, and others may have had a more malevolent motive than curiosity and unrecognized infatuation.

Bettina, stuck in her own totally self-centered twelve-year-old world-view, which included some aspect of attraction that made completely no sense to her, was in part trying to get Fleshy to laugh. In some respects, that thought elicits the most regret and guilt over her treatment of him. She looked at him a lot—well, gazed at him—and now in retrospect, realizes she liked how he looked.

But she never got him to laugh. The saddest part of all, in her shame-laced memory, is the half-smile. He never engaged in verbal combat; he would give a half-smile. One which you can't tell much about. The half-smile people give when they are not equipped to respond. The one she realizes now, fat people know very well, when you're not prepared to address a bully and hope with that half-smile they will just go away. That half-smile portrays some acquiescence that you get the joke and you are on board—just enough so that further clarification isn't needed. That's how Fleshy would respond.

He was a smart kid, and when he did engage Bettina, he never did so in a way that would point her out as a bully. He was always kind. But that says nothing about how he felt about the circumstance. Or perhaps it did. Perhaps kindness was armor.

Bettina doesn't remember any of the other kids teasing him, though he was the only large kid in the class. In fact, as she remembers it, he was the only large kid in the school. Perhaps that is why he didn't have any friends. Perhaps that is why no one else teased him. Perhaps that is all wrong. Perhaps all of Bettina's recollections are subjective and twisted with regret.

Besides, from the fact that, now, Bettina believes she was drawn to Fleshy in a romantic sort of way, that she found him cute, she might have had other hidden motivations for her behavior. She had become physically mature early, and that not only made her stand out at school, but it also caused her grief at home. As much as her mother had harped on her figure when she was Bones, a developing Bettina was at risk of getting fat. There were frequent warnings to be careful, that if you are not very, very careful, you are going to get fat—if you are not careful. And even discounting her mother, the messages in the culture were strong and clear. And twelve-year-old girls, especially ones who develop early, would be afraid of getting fat. Bettina's sister, ten years her senior, had been put on diet pills. As had most of her friends. They had been "sloppy fat." Sloppy fat was a favorite phrase of her mother.

It must have been a surprise to Bettina's mother when Bettina went from being too skinny to potentially too fat. It was definitely a swing of the pendulum; because she would lament the days when Bettina didn't eat enough and was just too thin, they seemed almost romantic now. But it was more complicated than that. There were four kids in the family—two girls and two boys—and a dramatic double standard. Bettina's mother didn't want the girls to be attractive, and certainly not to feel attractive. Her critiques of their clothing and hair could be vicious, and she was not otherwise a vicious woman. She later admitted regret for these condemnations, but at the time, preventing conceit was at the forefront of her mind—that was a sin. Humility and modesty were essential, and one should never, God forbid, seek approval from boys. This may appear to be in contradiction with her concern that the girls might become fat, but too much was always too much. It was as if the girls, in particular, should remain invisible.

There were several influences at play, but the primary one was religion. Bettina was raised strictly. Sexuality and even attractiveness were a threat to morality. The girls could not date until they were sixteen, and then only with a chaperone. The boys had more freedom, but were still expected to maintain purity. Should a woman in the neighborhood become pregnant out of wedlock, the judgmental clucking would never end. Shame was a pointed weapon, and cut deeply.

Though Bettina did disobey her mother, she did so with tremendous guilt. She lost her virginity at seventeen, sure there would be repercussions from God, and had she not feared God as she did, she would have lost her virginity earlier. There was also a sense of physical fear. Her mother had told Bettina horror stories about sex, about pain. Stories which were likely true from her mother's real experiences, but not stories that are wise to tell a young girl, unless you want them to be afraid.

It's not that the boys were encouraged to be handsome, and certainly not to have sex. They were taught about "those kind of girls." But they were allowed to travel farther away from home, including visiting their father after the divorce, who was living in sin with his girlfriend. Bettina was not permitted to do that, and as a result, her relationship with her father essentially ceased to exist.

Wanting her daughters to be thin was certainly not unusual, though in this case the motivation may have been. It is all too often that girls are told they will not be desired if they are fat. With Bettina, she was in essence told she would not be desired by God. Extra flesh might draw attention. It did with Bettina's friend Fleshy. She was attracted to his flesh, in her twelve-year-old way. The consequences of extra flesh on a girl could be dire, and she had already tempted fate by developing early. And, although Bettina did manage to get away with it, at least in the eyes of her mother, had the church found out she had sex out of wedlock she would have been disallowed, and not only from the church but potentially from her entire family.

There was, of course, frequent rebellion. Much drinking, which seemed to be a loophole in the teachings. And Bettina thinks perhaps her treatment of Fleshy may have been a bit of rebellion as well. The emotions were complex, and not really understood at the time, but Bettina, though not supposed to, stood out. That started long before her body blossomed, because her religion was one of no frills. During holiday or celebratory events, Bettina was told by teachers to drag her desk in the hallway and just wait, since she was not allowed to participate. Impossible not to be noticed. Fleshy stood out too; he was noticeable and Bettina noticed him. Her attempts to make him ever more apparent were indeed rebellion, as well as a rather clever bait and switch.

Fleshy was not the only victim of Bettina's public awareness of fat people. When she was maybe fourteen or fifteen, she was at a religious convention and was loitering with some of her girlfriends, as young girlfriends are wont to do. A woman passed by who was quite fat and Bettina puffed out her cheeks and tottered back and forth with her arms out to the sides, portraying fat in the way that people do when they want to state the obvious, but portray it as bad. She and her friends laughed as the woman clearly saw and heard—she was but a few feet away. This, of course, would have been bad enough if the woman was a stranger, but more than Fleshy, she was a friend. Someone Bettina liked very much, who had been kind and generous to her. Bettina's heart was broken by her own behavior. No doubt the woman had some feelings about the episode as well.

Bettina's getting caught mocking fat people is ironic for a variety of reasons, not the least of which is despite having been Bones, and her mother's strong warnings, Bettina grew up to become a very fat woman. Perhaps this is why she remembers these incidents so well. Not perhaps, actually. Clearly, it is.

Not only did Bettina grow up to be a very fat woman, but she also became a soldier in the fight for fat people, especially women, to appreciate their bodies as they are and to show those she calls civilians (the not fat) that not all large people are self-loathing, nor should they be. She feels that maybe those situations helped her to feel an obligation to make a difference in this regard.

There are aspects about her religious upbringing that Bettina still holds dear, though she has long since left the church. She has strict ideas about honesty, and in an interesting way, modesty. Not modesty about flesh, though it depends how one interprets the word. Bettina photographs nudes, fat nudes, unabashed and unashamed. Beautiful. But there is modesty in judgment. Modesty about shame—as in there should be none—for the body is, in whatever form, in essence, holy.

In her work, Bettina hears many stories. The people she photographs, mostly women, and mostly nude, often talk about their past, their childhood. They talk about their relationships with their mothers as they disrobe, as if peeling off their clothing also peels off the self-consciousness, the self-criticism, the self-doubt. For these fat people, the act of getting nude can be like a rebirth. Which makes it only more logical that Bettina would like to get in touch with Fleshy, now that flesh, and the fleshiest of it, is so integral to her contribution to the world, and in a sense, the essence of who she has become.

Bettina began to get fat when she married. Her husband was a big eater, and though not consciously, she attempted to keep up. She also suffered an illness that dramatically changed her metabolism, and the end result was a gain of 100 pounds. Interestingly, she did not have a lot of negative feelings about gaining weight. Perhaps it was all those years of being warned against vanity. Perhaps she had also always felt a kinship to large people. Whatever the case, she doesn't recall feeling terrible about becoming large. Though she did diet. It was the regular routine. Lose some, gain some more. She was among the first people in the United States to use fen-phen. There were only two doctors in the country experimenting with the drug at the time, and Bettina would drive four hours each way to see one. She lost 50 pounds so quickly she actually called the doctor for fear she might die from lack of eating. It was effortless, because she was so heavily drugged. It was also terrifying, and impermanent.

After many diets, and the pills, she stopped dieting. Gained back what she lost, and has stayed the same weight ever since. It's been about fifteen years.

Though she believes she had been a bully, she has never felt bullied for her weight. That's not to say no one ever mentions it. One day on a bus she almost fell on an older woman, who loudly exclaimed, "That's all I need, a 300-pounder falling one me." Bettina responded with, "You're very good at judging people's weight." The woman had nailed it. She has been stared at and clucked at, but for whatever reason, it doesn't hurt Bettina. She is not ashamed of her size. She has had a great deal of time to contemplate weight, what it means, and the reactions of others to it.

When she photographs her subjects, some of them are naked by the time she arrives, prancing around, full of pride and seemingly in love with their large bodies. Others have a much more difficult time. Some don't even show. She has heard every story, a great deal of damage caused by mothers and fathers, siblings, spouses, casual acquaintances, and coworkers, and even strangers. What they all seem to have in common is that their own attitudes guide their perception. Some people are much better at brushing off condemnation than others. Bettina seems to be a pro. Similar experiences can end in different results.

The truth is, Bettina did not feel guilty about Fleshy until after she got fat herself. In fact, she had forgotten him entirely. She realizes that while she handles those who mock or condemn her size well, if she had been bullied when she was a child she might be less forgiving of others, and herself. It really did take becoming fat for Bettina to find awareness and compassion when it came to weight. She didn't realize prior to that. It's not intuitive. Not in our culture. Bettina lives and works in a very politically liberal environment, where people constantly talk about fairness and rights. Yet when she brings up discrimination of fat people, fat activism, or fat rights, they often and honestly haven't the slightest idea what she is talking about.

It wasn't intuitive when Bettina bullied Fleshy, and without a doubt, now she believes she was a bully. Had she not become fat herself, she may never have realized that mocking and condemning a fat person is bullying. It's not intuitive. Not in our culture.

5

MORTAL COMBAT

Lisa has been in a lifelong battle, the enemy being her fat. She drags it through life, the arch nemesis layered entirely over her, in a conflict between her true self and the world. It is heavier than the actuality of the pounds because the weight of a rival is immeasurable, particularly when it is perpetually attached and seeming to cling for dear life. It's her or the fat. But there can be no winner, because she and the fat are the same. Lisa is her own enemy. She is in mortal combat with herself.

Lisa cannot remember a time when she wasn't overweight. She has seen pictures of herself as a toddler and she supposes she was normal then, but there is no place in her memory where she wasn't burdened by carrying extra, though that is to some degree in retrospect. Lisa didn't begin to perceive herself as abnormal until she was informed that she was. She wasn't exactly tormented; in fact, she interprets her experience with other children as having gotten off pretty easy. They merely teased her. That wasn't the worst of it, though. The worst was becoming aware of the separation of herself from others, that she was perceived as different from everyone else. That memory goes back as far as the first grade, or if she is being generous, perhaps the second.

It didn't help that her parents perpetuated the notion, although Lisa is quick to say they always had her best interest in mind. And undoubtedly, they did, but Lisa seems to carry this burden as if she deserves it, because when you are the burden, it is difficult to separate yourself from the blame.

So Lisa's parents would put her on diets. Nothing extreme, she says. They would restrict her portions at dinner, for one. And for another, they had firm ideas about some foods being good and others being bad. This led to guilt, because typically, bad was so good. She found those judgments much more difficult to shake than what the kids said to her. If a food was bad and she ate it, she, too, was bad. Though her parents didn't express it in quite that way, that is certainly how it felt—even though, as Lisa is quick to reiterate, her parents always had her best interest in mind.

Nevertheless, there are certain burdens that Lisa carries with her still, memories of being stricken by guilt because of food. There was the time at the county fair. Plenty of sights and sounds, but the one thing Lisa remembers most is the ice cream. After lavishing her with the forbidden treat, her father seems to remember just as Lisa is taking a bite: "You know, you really should not be having that," he reminds himself, his wife, and his seven-year-old daughter. Lisa's mother interjects: "No, it's okay, go ahead." That ice cream was no longer ice cream to Lisa. It was wrongness and shame. Her mother recognizes this reaction and berates her husband: "Look what you did now—she feels bad about it." And she certainly did. There was no enjoyment in that ice cream, or the collection of other random moments throughout Lisa's childhood where potential joy turned to perpetual pain, all for a taste of illicit food.

Lisa's parents were judging her. They were most probably judging themselves as well. But her parents' guilt did not assuage Lisa's shame. Her parents never openly criticized the way she looked, but the pressure to lose weight was there; the criticism was implicit. They claimed they cared primarily about Lisa's health—that was the message they intended to send, but Lisa interpreted those messages through the filter of the world she actually lived in. Through her peers, the starlets who were adored, the magazines she read, the television shows she watched, the wardrobe that she didn't fit. Nothing she gleaned from all that was about health. And although Lisa was given a sense her parents were primarily concerned for her health, it's not like they fully explained that logic. Perhaps they didn't think a seven-year-old would understand. Perhaps they didn't understand themselves. Instead, there was a pervasive idea that food was the culprit; it was inherently good or inherently bad. The skim milk had a property of goodness and the chocolate milk was innately bad, though she wasn't sure exactly why.

Eventually, of course, Lisa drew her own conclusions and made her own connections. It must be the sugar, and the fat. Sugar and fat are bad, and sugar and fat are in the chocolate milk. It wasn't innate; it was chemistry. And that realization could be applied to so many things. When sugar and fat were in the milk the milk became bad. When she drank the milk with sugar and fat, she became bad. Such is the maturation process of the dieting child; logic breeds contempt.

Lisa wasn't given special diet foods. In fact, she was treated exactly how the experts recommend. There were normal family meals, sit-down affairs with everyone together. She was given reasonable portions—everything in moderation. It wasn't unsuccessful, exactly, at least not when Lisa was young enough that her parents had full control of her food. She would lose some weight, but in doing so she gained a sense of discomfort. It felt strange to eat in front of her parents. There was always a sense of pressure; she was being observed. Whether Lisa's parents did continually monitor her isn't entirely clear, though it's not unreasonable to assume so. It doesn't really matter. Lisa felt it, and the real problems stemmed from her perception.

Now she wonders, sadly and futilely, about her parents' true motivations. Was health the primary concern—and since she wasn't in ill health, perhaps her weight would have just sorted itself out over time? And what about her mental health? If left to simply grow, would she have grown into her body, and her mind, with all the pieces in place?

To this day, Lisa is still trying to reestablish her "relationship with food," and her understanding that food itself isn't evil, that eating certain things doesn't make her a bad person. "I think my relationship with food has always been kind of out of whack, because you know, if I'm not going on an extreme diet, I am kind of aimlessly bingeing. There's no in-between." Lisa is only twenty-two. Based on the experiences of others who started dieting when they were six, about another twenty years should do the trick.

Lisa is an only child and grew up with both of her parents, who are still together. Her dad never had any weight issues, and if he wanted to lose 20 pounds, he just did. Her mother was a thin kid and also a thin adult, until after Lisa was born. But they believed the weight gain was due to the medications she was on. They also moved from a city, where everyone walked, to the country, where everyone walked to their cars. It was the perfect storm for weight gain, or so that was the observation. There were no other large people that Lisa knew of in her family line. Her mother's side was all thin and beautiful, terribly concerned with appearances, quite vain. Her father's side was just regular.

It seems as if Lisa's weight was in large part a reaction to her weight. A bit chubby, put on restrictive diets, and as soon as she had the freedom, she fought back with food. Lisa says she used food to soothe everything.

> When I was alone I would just eat, and eat, and eat. I would obviously hide this from my family, and once I gained enough weight, when I hated myself enough, I would join Weight Watchers or some other program, for as long as I could bear it. It was successful; I'd lose weight. Then something would snap and I couldn't do it anymore. It was a cyclical process through my whole life. Losing and gaining and losing and gaining. But why I put it on in the first place, I don't know. I guess it was that habit of using food as an emotional tool rather than a survival tool.

Or maybe it's because Lisa started dieting at six years old and was trained to rebel using food. Or perhaps it was biological. Though Lisa was taught certain food was bad, and she was bad for eating it, the way our brains and bodies respond to certain food is not a matter of rational thought. Nor is the process that predisposes us to store fat. That is not emotional dysfunction, it is cold, hard science, though our culture insists otherwise.

Lisa was indeed clinically overweight at six years old. She recalls the doctor referring to the BMI chart and pointing out her status. Sure, she was a chubby six year old. Maybe even a fat one. But a perfectly healthy child without a care in the world, or an eating disorder. Between the doctor's message and her parents' fear, the ball began to roll. Actually, is it was more her parents who pushed the ball. Her doctor did not suggest a diet. Doctors have never pressured Lisa to diet, interestingly enough.

Parents have fears, and understandably so. That is in large part their job after all. They wanted Lisa to be happy. They looked down the road and saw teasing, even bullying. And somehow, they sensed Lisa wasn't happy with her body, though there was both a chicken and an egg in that equation.

Through Lisa's childhood years, her dieting remained controlled by her parents and consisted of primarily monitoring portions and food choices. Her first commercial diet was her own idea. Lisa was about thirteen. She joined Weight Watchers, the first commercial diet of most dieters, and her mother joined with her. Although she doesn't remember all the details, she can't imagine her parents successfully promoting that idea if she wasn't on board. She was a bit of a surly teenager with a rebellious nature. She did what she wanted, and Lisa wanted to lose weight. She doesn't know all that much about her mother's feelings about her own weight—they didn't discuss it. But Lisa is aware that her mother seeks validation from her father, and her weight is a primary theme. Lisa also has no idea how her father feels about her mother's weight. He's not an affectionate type, a bit closed off emotionally, and he doesn't bring it up. But that doesn't say anything about his perception of his wife.

It was just prior to joining Weight Watchers that Lisa began using food to self-medicate, self-soothe, or whatever one chooses to call it. That was also around the time her parents started permitting her to stay at home by herself. Lisa didn't even realize she was doing it at first. Her mom would go out and Lisa would find herself alone in the house and the first thing that came to her mind was that it was time to eat. Then, it didn't occur to her that was unusual. She assumed everyone did it. It wasn't until Lisa was nearly seventeen that she stopped herself in mid-craving: Perhaps not everybody gets excited about being able to eat by themselves? Is that possible? She could only speculate.

By that time, she had organized various eating plots. She knew when and where she could get good grub. Her best friend was the daughter of a neighbor and Lisa would stop by on the way to school, just in time for breakfast. She had already eaten breakfast at home, but her friend's mom didn't know that and was more than happy to have a guest. This mom also served forbidden foods, making the caper all the more satisfying. Lisa found great enjoyment in being able to escape to that house of outlawed foods, or anywhere else they were available. And she took great lengths to conceal it. Her scandalous trysts with sugar and fat were fulfilling in more ways than one. Besides being delicious, they were a relief, a release of pressure, though in the end, when hating her body, she regretted them. But regret was not enough to dissuade her. Sugar and fat were far more powerful than regret.

At fifteen, Lisa came up with another weight-loss plan; she discovered weight-loss camp and was determined to attend. Lisa spent six weeks at the best fat camp in the country, one that nearly every fat kid eventually discovers and, if they can afford it, attends. As many fat kids do, Lisa enjoyed her time there. She lost about 20 pounds, but perhaps more important, she lived in this alternate universe where everyone was heavy. All the other aspects of teenage social life still existed—there were heavy pretty people, heavy nerds, and heavy cliques of all types—but everyone was heavy, and that made a world of difference. Plus, there was no thought about and no real need for self-control. They gave Lisa the food she was permitted and she ate it. The weight seemed to magically disappear. Fat camp was safe. It was a microcosm, a bubble, where everyone had fat in common, and in the scheme of social acceptance, being a nerd was one thing, and being fat was another. Though fat was the central theme of everything that went on in camp, it was also a non-issue. Dieting was like breathing—everyone did it.

Lisa never went back to fat camp after those six weeks, though she would have liked to. It was cost-prohibitive. But she also recognized a disturbing pattern. The kids would attend summer after summer, losing weight, and then gaining it back at home. As much as she liked the fat-camp bubble, it was also Lisa's first experience with skepticism in the diet industry. She felt jaded: "I realized why this thing would make money—people just keep going back every year." And indeed, they do.

It's hard for Lisa to say whether she believes there is a genetic component to her weight. She is inclined to say yes, because she wasn't always bingeing. When she was young, she ate normally, what her parents gave her, and she started putting on weight. Also, it seems from a physiological standpoint it is just harder for Lisa to lose weight than it is for some other people, like her dad. "Despite the fact that I don't feel like my body is where it should be, I can't imagine I'm genetically thin. I don't know, there are so many arguments for and against why people can gain weight, it's hard to say." *Arguments* may or may not be the correct term, based on science, but it certainly reflects our cultural attitudes. We spend a great deal of time arguing about the cause of biological processes.

Recently, Lisa began therapy for what the therapist classified as a binge-eating disorder. This does not sit altogether well with Lisa. She is aware of her eating patterns, her disordered eating patterns, but that label makes her uncomfortable. "I feel kind of funny saying I have a binge-eating disorder because people kind of look at you and basically think, 'So, you're a fat ass.' And I think, no, it really feels like a problem." Her bingeing began at around thirteen, and in what might be considered a classic representation of binge eating, it made her feel comforted, numb. "The experience afterward was not so good, but I admit, it was fun. Food was fun and the process was fun, but mostly it was soothing, and still is soothing."

The catalyst for therapy was, sadly, or perhaps luckily, ironic for a closet binge eater. Lisa started working in a candy store in her neighborhood; so quite literally, Lisa was in a room full of candy all day long. In Lisa's words, "needless to say," her binge-ing got out of control and she realized she had better figure this out. Whether therapy is helpful, Lisa says both yes and no. "It's definitely helping me understand a little bit more about why I do what I do, and how to control it a little bit. It hasn't helped my weight, but that comes down to more of me doing what I need to do and being responsible for what I need to work on."

She adds: "I've definitely always felt just bad about being fat. I can't get around it. I'd love to be one of those women who are just comfortable in their bodies and embrace themselves. But I've always equated my own fatness with being wrong in some way. I guess feeling guilty is a good way to put it."

And Lisa does blame her parents, she says, probably more than she should.

> I always look to them as the reason my eating patterns are so disordered. I wish I could go back in time and they would just allow me to listen to my body and figure out what it needs. I wish they had sat back and let me make my own decisions, at least to an extent. Obviously if a kid makes all her own choices about food he's going to eat candy for breakfast, but I do put some blame on them. Maybe I put too much blame on them. I feel like it gets to a point where the decisions I make are my own and I feel like what I did was my fault and not theirs. They trained me, in a way, but it was never a question of abuse. They were never intentionally harmful; they never said, "You're fat." It always came from a place of genuine concern and caring, and that's why I feel reluctant to point fingers. But

I guess they could be responsible even if they didn't mean to do what they did.

Lisa wonders if she is "addicted" to food, but feels conflicted about that too.

I think that maybe food addiction can be used as kind of a cop-out, where you say you are addicted to food. But to call it an addiction implies you need to stop, and we need food to live, we face it every day. On the other hand, there are times when I feel so out of control and so deeply bound to eating that I get to a point where I don't care about anything else. There's that emotional component and it's strong.

With my therapist we work on ultimately getting back to the point where I can intuitively eat and figure out what my body needs, just listen to my body and not emotionally eat. That's the biggest thing, trying to enjoy food and give myself permission to have what I want in an amount that I want, but not let the emotional component take over.

I feel weak in every way in regards to eating and weight and the idea that I just can't seem to shake this. Definitely.

But Lisa has stopped dieting.

It wasn't entirely a conscious decisions but I'm kind of at a point where I can't imagine going back to it. I did it for so long and just the thought of going through that whole process of degradation, control, and investing all that time and energy is exhausting to me, I can't imagine it. And not only can I not imagine it, I'm just at a point where I can't do it, I don't have it in me to go through with that again.

I want to set my relationship with food back to normal and sort of work backwards from that. It's obviously a much slower process, but it's one that I find preferable to just sort of slapping a big band-aid on the open wound and just hoping for the best. I realize that what I have been doing throughout my life, it wasn't working—that I clearly have a problem that is more than I happen to eat one too many slices of pizza, and that my relationship with food extends beyond just being absentminded in the way that I eat. I really wanted to address those issues in a psychological way rather than just trying to go back to the things, these unsustainable lifestyles—these diets have just been unsustainable.

Although Lisa still lives with her parents and they know she goes to therapy, they don't know, or at least it hasn't been discussed, that the therapy is explicitly for an eating disorder. "I haven't been ready to have that conversation with them because I find it so strange, and intimate, and painful, to talk about with them. So, it's sort of this unspoken thing." They still on occasion ask how the eating is going or whether she plans to join a gym again, and Lisa hates it.

I don't ever overtly respond negatively—it just kind of hurts my feelings because I wish they would just leave it alone. I find it frustrating, like if I have a snack and maybe it's not the most nutritious snack and my dad will say something, and I just want him to get off my back. I don't know why it is that I don't speak up. I guess that for a long time I felt that they were right and believed that, yeah, I am a shitty person for reaching for the cookies. When they say it, or I think they are saying it, it hurts even more. I can't imagine they would say it if they knew it hurt. But how can they not know?

Lisa feels judgment everywhere, from herself and others. "It seems like everyone is fat and I don't understand why there is so much stigma and hate around it. I guess I wish we could just eradicate the idea that eating itself is bad, the activity of eating. Also that certain foods are evil or forbidden. Just to get that stigma out of the way, be more understanding. Then maybe I could learn how to eat."

Lisa is in a war, with her body, with food, with society. She is in a war with her mind and her parents, and her behavior. With ideas others impose on her that she would like to rid so she can find peace within her own skin. It's not surprising she doesn't understand the stigma and hate. No one fully understands war—it is never entirely logical, and there are no winners in mortal combat.

PART TWO

PART TWO

6

THE SCIENCE OF FAT

An Interview with Dr. Emily J. Dhurandhar

There is more than a little controversy surrounding why people are fat and why they have difficulty losing weight and keeping that weight off. In discussions about weight, oftentimes the science is either misunderstood or completely unknown. In this interview, we are given essentially a primer on weight from the perspective of a clinical obesity researcher. Of course, this is not comprehensive, but it does bring to light some important issues of our time and helps to explain a good deal that is often misconstrued. Needless to say, on matters of perception, opinions will differ. Even on matters of science, there is often disagreement, and we are continually learning new information. Though as any scientist would agree, correlation is not the same as causation, meaning a link between two things does not indicate that one is definitively caused by the other. When there is a suggestion or tendency from a single study, that means there has been some link found in a particular set of circumstances. In other words, it appears as if it may be correct in that single situation, but one study alone is not proof. That is the nature of science.

Dr. Emily J. Dhurandhar has a PhD in human nutrition and is currently an Assistant Professor in the Department of Health Behavior at University of Alabama Birmingham as well as Chair of The Obesity Society Advocacy Committee. Dr. Dhurandhar is interested in both obesity research and advocacy. With her research, she aims to understand the regulation of energy balance and the biological and environmental factors that affect it in free-living individuals, with the objective of creating novel interventions for maintaining weight and for weight loss. Her advocacy efforts are focused on the impact of weight bias on both treatment and research in obesity.

* * *

Dr. Dhurandhar: I became interested in the topic of obesity when I took a nutrition class in college. During the class they talked about fat and fat consumption, particularly saturated fat, how it relates to cardiovascular disease and may be implicated in weight gain. We learned those basic principles, and I started to think about my mother and my father. It didn't seem like it could really be that simple.

My mother has struggled with weight all her life, she is an avid dieter, she's tried everything in the book. I got my undergraduate degree in nutrition, so I personally tried to help her several times with her weight loss. Then she became diabetic, which really amplified her weight gain due to the medications she's taking. Though she exercises quite often and tries to stay healthy, she still is very overweight. So I see her story as caloric restriction, dieting, and exercising. And then I see my father, who has always been as thin as a rail his whole life, and he has always enjoyed his food and has never had to make any attempt to control his weight. So I just couldn't accept the story I was getting in my nutrition class, that it's that simple.

When I went into graduate school I decided to study nutrition with a focus on metabolism—how our body utilizes nutrients, what factors regulate that, and how our body decides how much energy to expend. For example, whether or not some people are more efficient when they exercise, or if someone overeats, might that person be better at burning it off later than someone else who overeats. These kind of inter-individual differences were things that interested me.

During my dissertation work, my PhD, I studied a virus called Ad-36—it's an adenovirus, basically a common cold virus. It's actually not that well characterized because its symptoms are so benign, not severe, and therefore it's not well studied. However, if you infect animals with this virus, rodents and monkeys, it causes obesity. In humans you can tell if someone has had the virus in the past by looking for antibodies to the virus, and when we conduct that assay, the virus is pretty consistently associated with increased body weight and body fat mass. We have tried to look at this in detail, how is an infection able to do this? What we found is that in fat tissue everyone has something called preadipocytes, or pre-fat-cells, and if you put them in a petri dish and infect them with the virus, those pre-fat-cells will mature spontaneously into fat cells. So the virus seems to basically reprogram those cells to become bigger and gain fat. That is one possible way that the virus works and causes fat gain.

From this, I moved on to my postdoctoral work and have researched the kinds of exogenous factors that may cause obesity—such as infections, certain organo-pollutants, chemicals that act a lot like steroid hormones, and other factors of our modern-day lifestyle. For example, we all know that we're shifting toward a very sedentary lifestyle. We now do a lot of cognitive work, meaning we use our brains instead of our bodies. Studies show if you expend a lot of your brain resources in doing cognitive work, then afterward you will consume more energy (calories) than you really need to replace those calories you just expended. So it's as if we are not well programmed to regulate our energy intake in this modern work atmosphere of high cognitive demand. So that's another factor we don't typically think about, but it may really impact the way our body regulates food intake and our energy expenditure.

Those are just a few examples. I guess you could broadly say I am interested in trying to determine the kinds of alternative factors from our environment, our modern-day environment, that may perturb our energy balance, and might result in weight gain, or make weight loss very difficult.

Besides those exogenous factors, all those modern-day lifestyle factors, there are also internal things that we cannot control. For example, research suggests that excess weight may originate all the way back in pregnancy, so as you are developing in utero, there are factors from your mother that can actually transfer to you that make you more prone to weight gain as a child. So, even before you are born, there are things that can impact your body weight. And that's not an issue of willpower or personal choice. We are making progress, but there is still a great deal we don't know about how body weight is regulated and why some people are so prone to gaining weight in our modern environment and some people are not.

Q: Perhaps because of the research on obesity starting in the womb, doctors are beginning to prescribe dieting in pregnancy. That seems counterintuitive to what we know about healthy pregnancy, and also puts blame on the mother. If a woman diets in pregnancy will she prevent a fat child?

It appears to be a little more complicated than that, as usual. As far was whether or not a woman should or should not diet during pregnancy, we don't have a solid answer to that. We haven't done any rigorous carefully controlled studies to test that. There have been a few studies that aim to educate women about how to eat healthfully during a pregnancy and how to make sure they don't gain excess weight. But a lot of those educational programs have a minimal impact, if any, on weight gain in pregnancy. There is a very large trial funded by the National Institutes of Health that's ongoing right now that is attempting to prevent excess weight gain in pregnant women. I think the medical community in general would agree with you that severe caloric restriction during pregnancy is probably not ideal. However, I think they are trying to understand how a woman gains the optimal amount of weight during pregnancy. We actually do understand fairly well the appropriate amount of weight that should be gained during pregnancy—due to the infant, the placenta, and the extra body fat stores that are accrued for breast-feeding later. So how to ensure that the woman gains the appropriate amount of weight is what they are currently trying to understand.

I can understand the concern with blaming the mother. Just as it's not the fault of the infant that they are programmed a certain way because of the mother, it's also not necessarily the mother's fault. Really, I see excess weight as a chronic medical condition, and actually I would call it, in some cases, a disease. It would be like blaming her for transmitting any other disease to her infant. There is no issue of blame here. I think that's the wrong way of looking at it. Regarding the diet the mother consumes during pregnancy, it has been shown that a very high-fat, high-sugar diet may lead to excess fat gain in the infant and a large infant being born. So I would say it is probably optimal to eat a healthful diet when pregnant without severe caloric restrictions.

Q: The idea that consuming a very high-fat and high-sugar diet during pregnancy leads to a larger baby seems pretty logical. Does that mean the larger baby is going to be a fat person, or just that the baby ends up larger?

We know that if you look across populations at all different ranges of birth weight, the large-for-gestational-age infants and the small-for-gestational-age infants, both are at increased risk for being overweight as a child. So the thought is that the large-for-gestational-age infant is just programmed well for fat storage. The small-for-gestational-age infant, that infant when it's born goes through a very rapid catch-up growth phase, so it too is primed for weight gain. It's on both ends of the spectrum. These are, of course, tendencies, and do not necessarily apply to every child.

There are likely middle-weight infants that end up being over-weight later in life, and large and small infants that don't.

I would say that these factors I am discussing may predispose someone to be sensitive to weight gain. So for example, if someone is born normal weight and someone is born a very large infant, and as they grow up, they both are exposed to the same environment that encourages overeating and sedentary behavior, then the infant who was born large at gestational age may be more likely to gain weight in that environment than the child that was born at the normal weight. So these things may predispose you to a sensitivity to weight gain or even difficulty with weight loss. And this is just one of many possible factors that impact weight.

Q: Let's say a woman is overweight but eats a reasonably health-ful diet, not very high in fat and sugar, are those babies predis-posed to being fat?

Yes, that may be the case if they have a genetic predisposition to being overweight that is passed on to their offspring. It does appear, though, to also be linked to the intrauterine environment. There was a really well-done study that looked at mothers who gave birth before they had bariatric surgery and after they had bariatric surgery. So you can assume these women, before they had surgery, were overweight for some reason—it could have been from genetic predisposition, not eating unhealthily. Giving birth after bariatric surgery will still transmit that underlying genetic predisposition, but because of the surgery, they were able to lose weight. Those babies were born normal weight and have less of a tendency to be overweight in adolescence. Whereas, the babies born to mothers before the surgery are more overweight, and they tend to stay that way. That study suggests that even though the women may have a genetic predisposition to being overweight, just losing weight was sufficient to prevent transmitting that ten-dency to the child. That leads to the idea that something about the intra-uterine environment and the mother's current weight at the time of pregnancy has that impact on the baby.

Q: After bariatric surgery, people dramatically cut down on their food intake, generally eating around 1,000 calories a day. Also, there are commonly issues with nutrient absorption. Could it be that the smaller baby is a result of the calorie restriction or lack of nutrients, rather than the weight-loss surgery itself?

That is possible, we actually can't distinguish between the two, and it's really difficult to design a study to tease out those effects. It has been shown in a lot of animal studies that just the maternal diet alone is sufficient to impact the weight of the offspring. It most likely is a little bit of both, but we don't really have an answer to that question—it's a really good question.

Q: If underweight babies are predisposed to becoming fat people and the mother is consuming significantly fewer than the generally recommended number of calories for a healthy woman, much less a healthy pregnant woman, might bariatric patients be prone to having underweight babies?

Also an excellent question. Studies done so far suggest that bariatric surgery before pregnancy has better outcomes for the mother and infant. Actually one of the issues with studying bariatric surgery is that we don't have very good follow-up contact with bariatric surgery patients. Also, the amount of people who get surgery and then give birth is fairly small. So it's a bit complicated to study that question definitively, but so far, it doesn't appear that bariatric surgery makes women prone to having an underweight infant.

Q: Has there been any research on the difference between weight-loss surgery that rearranges the organs versus the lap band?

A lot of work has been done in the area comparing Roux-en-Y gastric bypass to the lap band for several things, like how well both work and how well both improve health in general. And one of the major findings is when patients receive that gastric bypass procedure, which as you said rearranges the digestive system, for whatever reason we see an almost immediate improvement in diabetes and blood-sugar regulation. Whereas, with the lap band surgery that just constricts your stomach, we don't see that effect at all. So that suggests that something about how the gut is arranged has an impact on the regulation on the blood glucose, and therefore, diabetes. That's one really interesting thing that has been found. And in general, the literature suggests that gastric bypass is more effective for weight loss than the lap band. It's marginally more effective, but it's more effective than the lap band. But lap band is reversible; it's not as invasive. I believe it also has fewer side effects and adverse events than Roux-en-Y gastric bypass.

Q: There has been a lot of discussion about a diabetes cure from the gastric bypass, which is fascinating. But that does not suggest that the gastric bypass is, overall, a safe or effective tool. It is merely saying that there's something going on in the gut, triggered by the change in the organ makeup, that impacts blood sugar. Do we know yet if there might be less invasive and potentially dangerous ways to get that same effect?

No, and that is correct, it does not speak to the surgery otherwise. There is a real flurry of activity trying to understand the mechanism so that we can develop a new therapeutic, less invasive way to create the same effect on diabetes, maybe a drug. So there are a lot of people researching that right now.

Q: Back to your research on the Ad-36 virus, can a person be tested for this; is it something a regular doctor can do?

Currently, we are able to test it in the lab, but a commercial standard approach to testing for it that would be used in a doctor's office isn't available yet. Dr. Richard Atkinson has started a commercial company called Obetech that will test if you have antibodies to the virus for a fee. At this point, what we know is it causes obesity in animals. It is associated with obesity in humans, but in science, you can't demonstrate that something is causal unless you can set up a very carefully controlled experiment. And unfortunately, with something like an infection, you can't do that experiment because it's unethical. So at the moment, this is a hypothesis that is reasonably well accepted now in the obesity field of research, but I wouldn't say that most medical doctors have even heard of it. I'm sure that some have now—it's gaining a lot of attention in the last decade or so. But it's not something your regular doctor can test for at this point.

Q: This is a virus. Once it is contracted is it something that could be potentially cured with medication?

In the case of Ad-36, based on what we know right now, one possibility is you could contract an Ad-36 infection and the virus would actively infect pre-fat-cells and cause them to grow, therefore causing your fat tissue to grow. That would happen at the time you are infected. It would then be cleared by the immune system from the body. The other possibility is it works like, for instance, the HPV virus that causes cervical cancer. That virus has a different method; once it infects your cell, it actually integrates itself into your DNA, so it stays with you, and certain things would trigger it to start replicating and have ongoing effects. Right now there's no evidence that an adenovirus like Ad-36 would insert itself into your genome and stay around as a latent infection. But it hasn't been really rigorously tested yet. That is one of the questions the Ad-36 researchers are trying to answer because it would have implications for the way it's treated. For example, if we know it has an ongoing effect, we can supply antivirals that actively stop the viral replication. Alternatively, vaccines against the virus could be used, so that no one gets it in the first place.

Q: Might Ad-36 be an explanation for the "obesity epidemic," that more of the population is getting fatter?

I think it is a possibility that it could be one of the factors. My inclination is to say that given what I know about all the potential factors that predispose you to weight gain, it is probably a cumulative effect of many things, which added together in the right combination has the greatest impact. Some of these factors we can track back as far as the 1950s or so, but it's bits and pieces. You can see correlations to many factors over time, but correlations are not causation, meaning there seems to be a relationship but we do not have definitive answers. For an example of a factor, there are organo-pollutants that act as hormones, PDBE for instance. We have data from breast milk in Sweden and you can see that the concentration of this chemical in breast milk has increased over time, since the 1970s. So we have some data that suggests such factors have been rising, and may have an impact on obesity rates. Before the 1950s, the data is limited. But we can start tracking it from here, so hopefully we can have a better understanding of all these things as we move on now.

Q: Why do you think kids are getting fatter as a population?

I think it is because of many factors—which one is most important, I don't know. One thing I have realized through my studies is that it is likely that the reason one person is overweight is not the same reason another person is overweight. There are different types of overweight that may result from different things. So of course, the increase in screen time and junk food in kids' diets and sugar-sweetened beverages—the general excess energy consumption and excess consumption of energy-dense foods in conjunction with school time and screen time and children watching

TV instead of playing—I'm sure all these things do prime children for becoming overweight. But I think a lot of the things we've discussed before, like maternal diet, genetics, perhaps this infection, there is also some evidence that the gut micro biome, the bacteria that live in your gut, might determine how you absorb food and how you process food. So I think all these things may come together to explain why some people, some children, are obese.

Q: So, whose fault is it that kids are getting fatter?

I don't think it's anyone's fault. I must say I have been trained as someone who looks at this problem from the perspective of your metabolism and your body, and yes, there are some personal choices that people can make, but that doesn't mean that the choices are easy to make, and it doesn't mean that they are practical to make, and it doesn't mean that your physiological makeup doesn't prime you to make certain choices, or make certain choices very difficult. The example I like to use is to compare body weight to height. As a person grows, if they get proper nutrition, they will grow to be a little bit taller. But nutrition only explains a certain amount of the variance in height from person to person, and actually, genetics also plays quite a big role, so it's a little bit of both, and I think obesity is very much the same thing.

Q: How much does dieting, and in particular yo-yo dieting, impact a tendency for people to become heavier in the long term than if they didn't diet?

I would say there is some evidence that frequent dieters tend to be more overweight than people who don't diet frequently. So just very generally speaking, that is a trend that is seen, but it's not clear if people who are frequent dieters are dieting because they're more overweight or if the frequent dieting is causing them to become more overweight. There's kind of a circular reasoning problem there. There is currently a study in mice being conducted that is seeking to determine if mice who constantly fluctuate in their weight live longer than mice who are overweight their whole lives. They are also comparing another group where mice start out very overweight but they lose about ten percent of their body weight and stay there. So they are doing all these different weight trajectories in the life span to see if weight impacts the life span. It should be very interesting to see what the results are, because again that's one of those things that are very difficult to test in humans.

Q: It is conventional wisdom that yo-yo dieting is unhealthy and that it results in many health problems. Is that accurate?

In general, the pattern that is seen is that when weight is lost, it's often regained within a year or so—a year to five years—depending on how much weight has been lost. Often the weight then increases even higher from where it started. So there does seem to be a creeping up associated with yo-yo dieting. Unfortunately, we don't know if, say, that same person never dieted, they would end up even heavier than they are after several dieting cycles, or if they would have stayed where they were. So unfortunately again, the answer to that question is not really clear and I know it is conventional wisdom, but we don't really know.

Q: It appears common that people who start to diet at a young age or diet frequently develop problems and eating disorders, binge eating, and emotional issues that contribute to weight gain. Do you also have to look at the psychology of yo-yo dieting?

When I made my statement, I was referring to metabolic health, cardiovascular disease, diabetes, and general weight and quality of life. But I wasn't speaking to the psychological health of an individual. I guess I can say that that's not really my area, but I can see how that may have an impact.

Q: It is also conventional wisdom that weight loss and obesity is simply about "calories in and calories out." How does a scientist respond to that belief?

That is a concept that comes from the first law of thermodynamics, which is energy can't be created or destroyed. So that means if you take energy in, it either has to be used or stored. However, while that is true, it does oversimplify things. Let's say, for example, if you are talking about macronutrient composition, there have been studies that show if you have diets with different macronutrient compositions, that can have an impact on body weight, and in particular, body composition. So some diets may prime you to store more fat than others in general. Most of that work is done in mice, so how translatable that is in humans is less clear. But you can imagine that the source of certain calories may determine how that calorie is used for a particular person, depending on their physiological makeup. And so it may be that the same number of calories is given to one person, and that same number of calories is given to another person, and maybe those two different people utilize those calories differently. That can have an impact on body composition.

There is also evidence that genetic factors can influence the energy expenditure side of the equation. There are really nicely done twin studies in which several pairs of twins were studied at a campsite, where they were completely supervised and isolated and had no chance to "cheat." It was found that twin pairs lost similar amounts of weight as a result of exercise, but the variation from twin pair to twin pair was much higher. That suggests that there is a genetic component to the response to exercise. In other words, some people are more efficient than others, and that has a genetic basis.

There are also other things that can impact your expenditure. Some people, when they overeat, recognize physiologically that they've overeaten and their brain tells them to increase their energy expenditure, and some don't. It's a component of energy expenditure that's now being studied more. When some people have overeaten, they start to fidget as a result. But some people do not get that signal; they just store what they have eaten. Yes, energy in equals energy out, but all the different things that impact the energy in and energy out determine your body weight and body composition, and that's a lot more complicated.

Q: Let's say somebody is obese and claims that they eat nutritionally, they don't overeat, they don't consume an excess amount of fat and sugar, and that they exercise regularly and sufficiently. Are they being dishonest?

Well, I would say no, they are not necessarily being dishonest, and it's kind of a difficult question. When someone says something like that, it's based on their own perception, and we know that people are not very good at judging their intake and what their intake should be. Both overweight people and thin people constantly underestimate the number of calories they've consumed in a day; it's a very consistent finding. People also tend to overestimate the amount of exercise they've had in a day. Everyone does that; it's not just overweight people. There's been a lot of work done in this area of weight loss—it's called *adherence*. When people go through weight-loss trials, a common curiosity is that some people lose more weight than others, even though this is supposed to be very carefully controlled. And what's found is that a lot of that variation can be attributed to adherence, so some people didn't stick to the diet as well as others.

But not all of it, and if you look at weight loss in mice and take adherence out of the equation, and everything is really well controlled—the environment, the amount of the food, the amount of exercise—there still is variation in the amount of weight loss. So I think it is plausible that a person thinks they are eating healthfully, and it may be that in fact they aren't eating a lot of fat and sugar, but they still don't have complete control over their weight.

Q: Is there a natural body weight set point, and can a person reach that with healthful eating and regular exercise?

The general notion is that your body should be able to maintain its weight, and it *should* know how much food you need to eat for how much energy you've expended. We understand fairly well all the different hormones and all the different pathways in your body that regulate your body weight and how much food to take in. But whether or not there's any kind of set point that is ideal, so to speak, and whether there is true homeostasis, we don't fully understand. Whether or not there is an actual set point, and whether you can train your body to be at that set point, is still disputed. There is a lot of good work that shows you can train people in the short term to eat fewer calories or eat certain food using different techniques such as smaller plate size and things like that. We've tested those things, and generally they work within a one-meal setting and sometimes over a 24-hour period. Unfortunately, we haven't tested those things over the long term. So whether or not your body can actually learn over time that you're eating well and reach a set point is not really understood.

Q: You mentioned that the body has a natural inclination to consume as many calories as it needs to maintain its current weight?

When we are in a healthy state and without any serious perturbations and stressors, that is theorized to be the case. But that may not be the environment that we are in. So when I say that, what I mean is when we take normal healthy mice and just feed them a reasonably healthy diet and don't expose them to a really obesogenic environment, they will maintain a healthy body weight on their own.

Q: Let's say a person weighs 300 pounds, is it their natural inclination to consume enough calories to maintain 300 pounds?

Yes, I would say if you eat less than you need to maintain your weight, you will be hungry, and you will eat more. Your body is programmed to fight weight loss. But it doesn't necessarily defend weight gain as well. If you overeat, what your body chooses to do with those extra calories is less clear. But we do know that in general, if you eat less than you should to maintain your current weight, you generally will get hungry and eat more.

Q: So basically, if for whatever reason you become overweight or obese, the body wants to maintain that state?

That's right, that's the way it's programmed.

Q: Whatever your weight is—let's say you weigh 700 pounds—to lose weight you still, technically speaking, have to starve yourself?

You have to eat fewer calories than it takes your body to maintain its weight, that's right. There is no other way of losing weight.

Q: And that is difficult?

It's extremely difficult, yes. There is no question about that.

Q: And it's difficult to maintain that over a period of time?

Yes.

Q: Can you explain why that is so difficult?

As you lose weight, certain changes in your body occur. If you reduce your number of calories and your body starts to lose weight, once it has recognized that weight loss is occurring, automatically your brain will reset your thermostat so that you don't expend as much energy. At your new lower weight your body is trying to preserve its mass, so your normal resting energy expenditure goes down. That means that to continue losing weight you have an extra deficit you have to account for, because now your body is not expending as much, so you have to reduce your calories even more to still be in negative energy balance and continue to lose weight. That kind of compensatory response from your body automatically makes dieting more difficult. There are also hormones in your body that are meant to inform your brain as to the level of body weight that is there, and as you lose weight, pretty consistently your hunger hormones will be ramped up. In general, you're primed to want to eat when you are in a negative energy balance state.

Q: Is that what one refers to as the metabolism?

"Metabolism" refers to a lot of things, but in reference to weight, it refers to the accrual of energy and the expenditure of energy. So when I say metabolism I am specifically referring to energy metabolism, and that's speaking very broadly.

Q: You talked about a number of factors, particularly the brain changes to accommodate the lack of energy consumption. Is that essentially what metabolism is when we're talking about losing weight—when we say the metabolism is slow?

Yes, that's right, it's kind of the layman's term for it.

Q: Is a person born with the innate desire to crave foods that are most healthy for them, and it is merely our society that perpetuates cravings for fats and sugars?

I don't personally know of any scientific evidence to support that concept. I will say that when you are born, you are very primed to seek out certain tastes, so you know that sweet and salty is good, and you can identify that. So there are some basic tastes that you will seek out as an infant that are programmed.

Q: From a biological perspective, can a person train himself to crave healthier foods like vegetables, rather than foods high in fat and sugar?

It appears we are very well programmed to overeat, rather than eat what we're supposed to. If you think about it, it makes sense in a world where famine was common, and the fattest person was the most likely to survive. Though times have really changed, we aren't necessarily well equipped for our current environment. We are programmed to seek out energy-dense, sweet, salty, fatty foods. Those foods highlight reward circuits in your brain, and eating that food is a very reinforced behavior. If you think about someone craving broccoli, that may be achievable with a certain mental state, but I wouldn't say that that's something everyone could achieve. And it's certainly not something that I think your body would program you to do. It doesn't make sense; energetically, broccoli is not a very valuable food to your body.

Q: What do you think we should do about the "childhood obesity crisis"?

I think that probably the most important thing we can do is to recognize that the childhood obesity epidemic is a very serious problem that cannot be boiled down to blaming, really, anyone. I think we need to take it seriously as a medical condition that we need to research further, and we need to treat as a medical condition. It's, of course, natural that conventional wisdom would come up (like calories in and calories out), because we don't necessarily have a better explanation. But I strongly believe that the most important thing we can do is treat it seriously, and to recognize as a society that it is not necessarily going to be fixed with just fruits and vegetables and PE in schools. In fact, in the school-based studies that used those techniques, sometimes they have success in increasing fruit and vegetable intake or increasing activity level in kids, but the overall impact on body weight on children is minimal. I think there are good reasons for that and it would help if we recognized it as a very complicated problem and move forward from there.

Q: What do you think of putting children on diets?

I think that if a child is gaining so much weight that he is showing co-morbidities like high blood pressure, hyperlipoproteinemia, and high blood sugar, that in some cases it can be appropriate to place a child on a weight-reducing diet, because that is the only tool we currently have if a child's health is in immediate jeopardy. But in general, it would be best to simply encourage healthful habits in children, and not have the focus be on weight, but rather have the focus be on health—leading a healthy, responsible lifestyle—and then understand and accept that the focus on health may result in different things for different people. A child that is slightly overweight, that has a pre-pubertal fat spurt, I don't think a diet is necessary or appropriate for that. As far as we know at this time, dieting in children should be reserved for those who are really in trouble.

Q: Using myself as an example, I was put on a diet at six by my pediatrician. I was a chubby kid but I was perfectly healthy. I continued to diet for thirty years. My story is typical. A chubby kid gets put on a diet by a doctor, and it starts a lifelong pattern of weight gain and loss and eating disorders and psychological issues. So in my case, do you think my doctor made the right decision?

Your pediatrician most probably did what he thought was best. For a child such as yourself that we know is overweight, the chances of that child becoming overweight later in life are pretty high. A lot of people are treating kids for obesity as a preventative thing. I think that's a common mentality. At this point, that may be the best approach that we have, but that's not to say we shouldn't try to do better, or that it's necessarily a good solution. I'm sure many people have the same story; it's a long, losing battle, really. The medical community is finally beginning to recognize that weight loss with just diet and exercise is very difficult for most people, and maintaining it is even more difficult. As a society, we should consider the cost/benefit ratio, because I know the psychological cost can be quite damaging.

Q: What is the most important thing people should know about how we become overweight and how we lose weight?

The most important thing that I could get across is that this is really complicated; obesity is a really complicated disease and it needs to be seen that way. We need to help people understand the complexity of it, so that people such as yourself don't face blame and stigma, and so we can move forward with the full support of society and the medical community to treat it more effectively.

Q: What is your take on the American Medical Association classifying "obesity" as a disease?

Recently the AMA classified obesity as a disease. Although not all patients with a body mass index (BMI) above 30 that fall into the "obese" category have co-morbidities related to obesity, and obesity is a heterogeneous condition, this is a first step to reducing stigma in the medical examination room and treating obesity as more than an issue of willpower and personal responsibility. Because not everyone with a BMI above 30 has co-morbidities, I hope eventually we can come up with an improved definition and clinical markers that signifies a fat-related disease state. There is evidence that fat tissue can be "healthy" or "unhealthy," and although the health of fat tissue is correlated with the amount of fat tissue (and thus with BMI), we still need better ways to distinguish individuals with and without a fat-related disease state. There are people actively researching this.

Nonetheless, there are several important implications of this decision. Classifying obesity as a disease, or a health condition that may be, at least in part, due to circumstances beyond an individual's control, will open up the discussion to address it seriously and to persistently pursue all potential treatment options. It will help to overcome that barrier of blame and shame that currently occurs in the medical examination room. It will also force health insurance companies to consider covering its treatment. Additionally, treating it in a formal and standardized way will help evaluate and improve current standards of care. Lastly, classifying obesity as a disease will eventually create a medical support system for the treatment of obesity, which will, importantly, educate the public and put an end to the quackery that preys on obese individuals who are trying to lose weight every day.

Q: In large part because of the many things you have discussed, there is a movement to focus on health rather than weight. In some circles, it is called HAES (Health at Every Size). This does not suggest everyone is healthy at every size, but rather the more productive focus is a healthy lifestyle rather than the number on the scale. The goal is to be physically and emotionally well, though not necessarily thinner. From your experience, do you believe that this is a wise objective?

Although body mass index is a useful starting point to evaluate health, evidence suggests that it is not always a very precise indicator. Thus, an emphasis on overall health and healthy habits is a sensible approach.

7

BETWEEN A ROCK AND
A DEFENSIVE TACKLE

"**Y**ou don't want any other kid to go through what you've gone through."

That's Ben. He's eleven years old, and he's gone through quite a bit for a boy of eleven. That he doesn't want any other kid to go through it too speaks volumes, not only about the kind of kid Ben is, but also about what it's like for any kid to be a fat kid. He is just the nicest, most thoughtful boy, and that's a testament to his mother, because whether or not she took the road you would have taken, there is no questioning her commitment to the happiness of her son. And he is happy. He wasn't as happy, though, when he was fat.

Benjamin loves football, and chocolate volcano cake. His drive is more toward the field, but it's hard to say if that was always true. It might have been, if people had allowed it. This all started when Ben was just a boy of eight. He began to get a little round about the edges. Everyone in the family is on the heavy side. The women are what you would call plus size, and the men, big guys. Ben was born to be large—it's in his genes. One might think that would work well for a boy who pretty much lives to play football, but not when you're eight. The rules are very different then. And in fact, as Ben tells it, it's not all pep squads and glory for the big guys playing grown-up football either. A big guy is never the quarterback.

By nine, Ben was a full-fledged fat kid. Although his mother wasn't entirely aware of it, his life at school was a living hell. He was teased unmercifully. "They'd say it in the hallway and classroom. They'd call me stupid and fat. Fat, stupid, ugly, bad words, the f-word, the b-word, all those, all the ones, f-you, fatso, f-u-c-k, b-i-t-c-h." The fat kids were a dumping ground, for emotional aggression and leftover lunch. Anything the other children didn't want at lunch was presented to the fat kids—"They'll eat anything." He had a few friends, and they didn't care what size he was, but outside that circle their opinion didn't matter much—in the social scheme of things their only value was in being the objects of ridicule. Whatever other hierarchy existed in elementary school, the fat kids had a spot to hold up: the bottom.

Ben frequently came home crying; even with the frogs and snails and puppy-dogs' tails of which he was made, little boys have a breaking point. Still, he tried to fight back. It was school policy to report bullying to the teacher, and Ben did. He did so often—so often, in fact, that during his fourth-grade parent-teacher conference his mother was informed Ben was an unrepentant tattletale. So much for zero-tolerance on the bullying front. That summer Ben had the opportunity to go to fifth-grade camp. His parents pleaded with him: "It will be the best experience of your life." Staunchly against it, Ben caved and went anyway. He had actually lost a bit of weight by then, and hoped his smaller-ness might make him immune. Not so—the previous year had been torturous enough that to the now ten-year-old, any insult was kryptonite.

The first night of camp Ben's parents got a call. They were to pick him up immediately! Camp did have a zero-tolerance policy. That day, a kid smugly walked up to Ben and made his power move: "You're fat, and ugly." Ben hauled off and decked him. In fact, Ben pummeled the kid, and was unable to make himself stop. He beat that kid in the name of every other kid who ever called him fat. He had never hit anyone before. He doesn't even really remember the incident. It was as if, he says, he saw red. Just recently having been reprimanded for tattling, hungry from dieting, and the best experience of his life starting out as a brand-new entrance to hell, Ben's little-boy makeup could comprehend no other option. Not that it was a calculated move.

"All of a sudden he said it and I just wasn't myself. I went at him and I couldn't stop. It was bunched up inside of me and it just came out. He said fat and ugly, why are you so fat and ugly? I just railed on him. It did kind of make me feel better because I just let all my anger out." Ben's mom says, "He was crying, he was hitting him and crying at the same time, and they had to pull him off because he couldn't stop. So all of that was just coming out. I've never seen it before, or since." And Ben was summarily dismissed from camp. Not for nothing—the counselor privately told Ben's parents he wanted to sock the kid too. Not for nothing.

Prior to starting camp Ben's mother had attempted to put him on a diet. It seemed like the reasonable thing to do. It seemed like it would be easier to change her son than all of society. And the truth is Ben didn't like being a fat kid; besides being teased, he couldn't run as fast as his classmates, he got tired more easily, and there were restrictions on playing football. The latter was the clincher, football trumped all. So Ben's mom tried to help him reduce his food. She says that, after all, he did eat a lot of it. If it was available he could down three pieces of pizza, two brownies, a cupcake, and a slice of pie. She would tell him, "You can't eat all of that, it's too much." And Ben would respond like any kid being told he couldn't do what he wanted to do: He had a fit. But it was deeper than a tantrum. Ben felt punished and betrayed. Other kids got to eat the good stuff, why not he? He would scream at his mother, "You hate me, you're so mean to me, you don't want me to have anything." Regardless of intention, she became the bad guy. They would fight. Their relationship suffered and they were both miserable. "They come to us crying at first because they're fat, and then we try to help them and they're crying that we hate them. It's a no-win situation for parents, I can tell you that." Also, Ben didn't lose any weight.

The question of whether to give up or keep going was answered, not by bullying children or even by their own desires. It was answered by desperation and the city in which they lived. By circumstances that truly left Ben's mother without the option to do nothing. There is a point where the unfortunate becomes the absurd, and Ben was kicked over that goal line. Touchdown. Spike! It was because of football.

Ben loves football. He lives for football. And as soon as he could, he joined the football team. By age nine he was a member of the city-run league. It's fair to say that every boy who ever lived in that city at least considered playing in the league. Where Ben is from, everyone is into football. It's probably like that where you live too. And since it is, you already know that football is forgiving, in that different players are different sizes, and different-sized players have different roles on the team. In football, being a big dude is not necessarily a bad thing. You won't be a quarterback, but you certainly can have an important role throwing your weight around.

"The really small kids are quarterbacks, runners, or catchers. The fat kids were on the line. I was an offensive kid, so I would usually just lay on my guy and he'd go down. I did play defense a little bit and it was harder because I was slower." The problem for Ben was that, even in tackle football, permission to full-on pummel doesn't begin until high school. At nine, and for the next five or so years, the player's weight has an enormous impact on not only the position they play but also on whether they can play at all.

That is not uncommon. It is not uncommon that the boys, like Ben, have to be weighed before each game. It is not uncommon that they are told not to eat before weigh-in, have to strip down to their skivvies, and have their weight monitored by their own coach and the other team. "They have one weighing session where all the kids go at the beginning of the season, and if you are close or over the cutoff you have to keep weighing. You have to go into this trailer and strip down to your underwear as a fat kid. They weigh before each game and sometimes during some practices—two practices before the game just so they know if you're safe or you need to work." For better or worse, this is not uncommon in competitive sports.

It is also not uncommon that the kids who have not made weight are treated very differently. For instance, during practice, instead of learning plays and practicing the game, they run. They run and run. They run until they can't run anymore, and then they run farther. Although Ben had to do this, he certainly wasn't the first. Ask any fat kid football player (or grown man who was a fat kid football player) if they ran during practice instead of actually practicing, and chances are you will find it's a time-honored tradition. They suck it up. That's football.

Mind you, this was happening long before the "childhood obesity crisis" existed. The running is not for health, it has one sole purpose: making weight at the next game. Perhaps it has a second purpose, but not one that gets printed in the newsletter. That would be: punishment for not making weight at the last game.

What may or may not be historical is that the boys who don't make weight before a game can only play for part of the game—in this league, three plays in each half. They get benched the remainder. There are theoretically rational reasons for this. For instance, if a small boy is up against a big boy, the small boy might get hurt. Fair enough. But then why three plays? It's safe for three, but not for ten? Is three a magic number or are they randomly playing the odds? Or perhaps they are concerned for the large boy's welfare—an entire game could be too strenuous for a large boy. Except that has nothing to do with it. How would they explain all the running? Plus the boys have all been medically cleared. And, well, no one outside this sentence has ever considered that notion. Besides, Ben wasn't too tired to continue, he was climbing out of his pads to get on the field.

So, boys who don't make weight play for only a portion of the game. Perhaps not everywhere, but certainly in Ben's league. However, at least in Ben's league, and it seems most everywhere else as well, there is no well-planned grand scheme for when the big boys can play and when they are benched. They go in for a certain number of plays; the coach determines which. There is no consulting with the opposing team to match up like-sized boys so that no one gets hurt. In fact, probably the opposite is true—probably using bigger boys against smaller ones is a tactic. Probably it's time to throw in the fat kid when the puny boy on the other team plays. This is still tackle football. And the goal is still to win.

At any rate, as is the rule, Ben played a limited amount of time per game, as determined by the league, when his coach said so. For the rest of the time he watched. On Ben's team, there were usually about four boys in the same boat in any given season. If a boy was too big, he got sent up to junior varsity or varsity with the older boys. But that wasn't a bonus. He wouldn't have the skills of those older children and would warm the bench permanently.

While not playing was frustrating, receiving no good explanation for the allotted play time was infuriating. They asked. Of course they asked. Either no one knew, or no one was telling. Perhaps a little of both. Also not uncommon. Just ask any fat kid who plays, or played, football. "It didn't feel really good, and I would feel bad about myself. Sometimes I would get angry. I kind of had it inside, I never really said anything. I was angry inside. I couldn't do anything about it."

Though most of this is not uncommon, there was an unusual aspect to the way Ben's city league dealt with the fat kids. These boys had a name—they were called the "X Men." Why they were originally dubbed the X Men is not clear; it may simply have been practical. The X Men, you see, were branded with a big *X* on their helmets. All the X Men had the letter *X* embossed in tape, right smack on their heads, so everyone watching—the coaches, the players, the people in the stands—knew who the X Men were. They had a scarlet, or at least a duct tape, letter. Certainly that made it easier for the X Men to be identified, but football had already addressed the concept of identification with names and numbers on the uniforms. So the necessity of the *X* on the head of a fat boy—who was clearly fat because his body was shaped that way, and even if somehow he magically didn't appear fat he had his name and number on his jersey—served no actual functional purpose. Unless of course the purpose was one excluded from the rule book: humiliation.

And if humiliation was the goal, that X was extraordinarily effective, because Ben was mortified. His mother was furious. The league was mystified. And the practice of marking the X Men went on—had been going on—for a long time. Until Ben's mother started talking about it publicly. That is not uncommon.

Oh, and as this was a city team, so all the team members paid to play, which is only significant if you enjoy grotesque irony. Not ironic at all, just despicable, is that another aspect of being one of the X Men is that the city team forced food restrictions. When the team went out for pizza to celebrate a good game (or what have you) the X Men weren't allowed to eat. Those nine-year-old boys sat in the pizza joint along with their mates, and watched. It's a wonder there wasn't a riot. It's no wonder Ben would come home crying.

> It wasn't good because everyone on the team, and the other team, they all knew I was a bigger kid and I only get a certain amount of plays because they marked us with the X on the back. It was not good knowing a whole bunch of people are watching you and they know that you're fat. I wanted to quit sometimes. I wanted to cut school a little bit because it got pretty bad there. I didn't want to go to school because there are kids there being mean and calling me fat and all that. Sometimes I said I was sick so I could stay home.

The obvious dilemma for Ben's mom was that even if she could stir up enough trouble to have these policies changed, her son would pay the price. Ben was damned if she did and damned if she didn't. It's not like any of this was a secret. The coaches, teammates, and parents would all know Ben, the fat kid, was responsible for this mess—one of the group (fat kids) that for generations just sat quietly by and tolerated it. And even if Ben's mom ended up a hero, no nine-year-old wants a hero for a mom. He just wanted to play football, without shame, and have a celebratory slice of pizza as part of the team.

Since there was no good solution, Ben's mother picked the better of the bad. She decided she had to find a way to help Ben lose weight without destroying him or the family. "It's hard enough for us as adults to try to eat right and understand what it takes to be healthy; it's that much harder for children." After many sleepless nights and exhausted days she came up with a plan. Ben loved money. Some people are just born to be investment bankers or MBAs, and Ben is one of them. "This kid, he would go to his sister's soccer games with a bag of caramel corn and he would go around to all the parents and sell it by the handful for a quarter, and come back with half a bag and a bunch of quarters. He's always been driven by money. I knew I had to come up with some kind of way to tie eating healthy with money."

She didn't want to pay him for pounds, which has certainly been done before, and is generally a miserable failure for a host of reasons. And it wasn't so much that Ben wanted money—he was interested in money. He found the concept of money and money exchange, business in general, fascinating. And he could sell a bridge to any reluctant buyer. Ben's mom capitalized on that and came up with a game that, not unlike the concept of Weight Watchers points, involved a swap of calories for numbers. But Ben couldn't care less about Weight Watchers points, and they made no sense to him anyway. Why is a cookie worth two points? Why two? But if a cookie is worth two hundred dollars, that's something.

Ben's mother devised a system (she never called it a diet) in which every calorie was worth a dollar and Ben was given a certain amount of "fun money" each day to spend. "I liked the money thing because I just love, love, love money," said Ben. His mom explains:

So if it was recommended he had 1,800 calories for that day, I would give him 1,800 dollars in fun money in the morning. Ben could eat what he wanted, but he couldn't eat more than he could afford. He could still enjoy some of the things that kids like, like a slice of pizza. Pizza is 300 calories, so instead of eating three or four pieces of pizza, he would pay me for one piece—he would give me 300 dollars of his fun money. But all fruits and vegetables were free, so he'd say, "I'll make a huge salad and have an apple with my slice of pizza." He wasn't being deprived of the foods that he enjoys, but he was eating less of them because he was more aware of how much they cost, and that's how it worked for him.

Even things like going to the store and wanting a Snickers candy bar, well, that would cost almost 300 dollars, so he would buy sugar-free candy with zero calories. We weren't trying to tell him he couldn't have the things he wanted; we were trying to make choices a more positive experience for him. You can have those things, but you can have them in moderation, because they add up quickly. He could also save up a percentage. If he didn't want to use all of his 1,800 dollars he could save up to 20 percent that day. We didn't want him under-eating either, so he had to spend at least 80 percent of his money each day, but he could save the rest for the weekend, for birthday parties, or if he wanted, something special. Or he could put it into a savings account and build it up for rewards.

Ben learned the concept of calories, how much was in each food, and began to balance his food intake according to his wallet. Ben was surprised that if he ate three pieces of pizza he spent half of his daily funds, so he opted for one piece instead. Ben's mom was surprised that he not only didn't resent the plan but he actually enjoyed it. He found it interesting, and fun. Also, he lost weight. Ben wasn't ashamed of this new regime (which they called a game); he was proud of it. He discussed his game with friends, if they were interested to listen, and he says their response was always positive. He began to have such a keen grasp on the calories in food that after a time, he didn't need the money anymore and just ate the right amount by instinct. If he would gain a few pounds he would ask his mother to bring out the dollars and they would tighten up the rules for a while.

There are all kinds of happy endings to this story. Ben is no longer one of the X Men. All X's have been removed from helmets, and pizza for these players is optional rather than forbidden. Ben is proud of himself; he feels that he can run faster and longer and plans to take up baseball as well.

> Now I feel much better. I was a captain last year so I might be one this year too. Now I play hiker, left tackle, right tackle. I play a whole different bunch of the spots on the line. I play offense and defense. I do a lot of different stuff now. Last year I did better, so I was the line captain, I had to make sure my line was doing good. I would be on the line and I would hike the ball, be left tackle and all that. Before each practice, we all run a lap around the field, and the field is humungous because we have four different fields with four different teams playing, or five, and we had to run around the entire thing. I used to always come in last. Now I'm middling up, so it's better. And not one kid in my school bullies me anymore. I have lots of friends. I like going to school better. School is still school, but, at least I have friends.

On the other hand, fat kids still get weighed in their shorts, run during practice, and play only part of the game. But the city seems sufficiently uncomfortable about any extraordinarily humiliating practices.

Ben and his mom have also gone into business together. They have taken the "fun money" concept and have turned it into games that they had professionally produced and that they work to market. They even make public appearances together. Ben feels no shame. Doctors, nutritionists, and school officials give the games high marks, and kids who play the games seem to enjoy them—at least the one game where food choices are theoretical and they don't have to actually monitor their pizza. Whether the fun money concept would work for different kids when it comes to real food is unknown. This was an idea built for Ben, and it seemed to work very well for him. He also has an extremely thoughtful and attentive mother who spent a great deal of energy throwing away the bad ideas, which may be a huge part of the success of this project. Ben is only eleven now. No one has a crystal ball that will see his future. But if you are looking for a kid who is proud of himself and his accomplishments, look right here.

As for Ben's forthcoming life with fat, he is fighting genetics. He comes from large-size people on both sides. They all acknowledge that for this family, weight is something that will always have to be watched; they are built to carry a lot of it.

> I just think that our whole family, my mother and my sister, they're all size 20, 24, my husband is six foot tall, 300 pounds. I've always dealt with weight, our whole family, it's set against us to be overweight, so I think if Ben looks at food, he gains weight. It's just unfair because this kid, now today, will go out with his friends and will order a grilled chicken wrap or something, and he'll order a salad instead of fries, and still he's not skinny. He's not fat anymore, but he's not skinny. His friends eat the Big Macs, French fries, and milk shakes, and they're twigs, so it's just—I think it's how you're built. When he was around eight, he started gaining—I don't know if all of a sudden he started eating more, I just think he was going to be a big kid, if he didn't make an effort, and to this day if he doesn't watch himself he gains weight fast.

Ben says,

I was upset that I was a fat kid. I always came home crying because I got bullied. It's not a good thing, being fat, for a lot of reasons. Skinny kids get to eat more, and they always get to do more things, and get more popular. They get more popular, they get more friends. They are usually starters on the football field and usually have a lot of perks over bigger kids. I had some friends when I was fat, they didn't really care if I was bigger or smaller because I was their friend. Other kids gave me a hard time. Usually, they were strangers and kids in my school who were popular, and skinny. Also the other kids were faster, they always did better than me, I didn't feel like I was good.

It's weird because I see a lot of my friends who are super skinny, who are a twig, they eat like two pretzels, pizza, and all this. At my last school, this one kid, he was so skinny he could eat three lunches each day, and still, he was so skinny. It just doesn't make sense. I think it's just how they're made. You can't really help how you're made. You can try, but you still—if you stop trying you're gonna be however you're made. I'm gonna try, I'm gonna have a bad day every once in a while, go have something really bad. But then the next day I will try and watch what I'm eating, so I guess I'll still watch because I know my family is usually bigger, so I have to watch all the time.

Perhaps most poignant in this whole story, though, is Ben's circumspect attitude about fat people—both himself and others. He has lived on both sides of the fence. It is not uncommon for people who have lost weight to have a negative perception of those who haven't. ("If I could do it, then . . .") And Ben is just a little boy, so he may or may not have the capacity to parse out the complexities of the issues. And indeed, he feels both very empathetic and also just a little judgmental, though primarily he cares about justice.

When I see a fat kid I usually think that I should be nicer to them because I know what happened to me when I was bigger. I don't want that to happen to anyone else. I never think anything bad about that kid. I know they might feel better if they started working out and eating a little better, but I never say, "Fat—ha-ha." Some of my friends are fat, on the football team and in school. I'm kind of a shy kid so I don't usually say things about losing weight, but if they came up to me and asked me or said something, I would probably tell them about what I did and see if they like it.

I think thin kids are mean to fat kids because they think they are better than them, just because they are a little skinnier and they can probably do a little more, so they think they are better. Maybe their parents taught them that, if when they play sports they said things like, "You came in behind the big kid—work harder, work harder." Kids might feel that way themselves too. I sometimes see something on TV, like the fast kid runs past all the bigger kids and everyone cheers. The fat kid always comes in last, and that is kind of unfair.

When asked why he thinks kids are fat, Ben is also a pragmatist.

People are coming up with new tasty things that taste really good, but are a lot of calories, like volcano cakes, chocolate volcano cakes, and all that, and they're just really tasty. Everyone just has to have them. Who could deny?

You just have to keep trying and trying, if you try and try you're probably going to succeed. But some people try to lose weight and still have a hard time. You don't really know unless you know them. But even if you don't try to lose weight, or don't succeed, never think that you aren't as good as anyone else—everyone is equal. Fat kids shouldn't think that just because a kid's skinnier and they are more popular, don't think he is better than you. I try and watch, sometimes I just forget about everything and I don't keep track and I look at the scale and it's up another five pounds, or six, or seven, or eight, or nine, or ten, but then I know I've got to get together again and keep trying.

As for Ben's mom, she says,

If it weren't for that stupid X we probably never would have done this, so we see it as a blessing. There were three suicides last year in the middle school and it makes me so sad to think my son could have been one of them. He hated life and hated school—what would have kept him from taking measures if it continued? Kids can be so mean. The whole world is mean; I don't know how we are going to change it. I would rather focus on the person who is being mistreated, you have to find ways to make them feel better. As my son says, even if you're overweight, no one else is better than you.

8

STARVED

Certainly not everyone who spends their formative childhood years in a prison camp ends up with body image issues. But it happens.

Leigh was born in California but raised in Las Vegas. Growing up in Las Vegas is many things you would expect it to be, and many things you would not. While the adults were living 24-hour lives working in the gaming industry, Leigh was riding her bike, playing ball, swimming, climbing trees, searching for secret hideouts, and riding a minibike, unicycle, and pogo stick. She had all the baseball and football gear a girl could dream of. She grew up basically doing everything a quirky tomboy could do in the vast terrain of the desert on the outskirts of the neon city. If Leigh wasn't throwing a ball, she was riding on wheels, and if not that, climbing, jumping, running, or splashing. It would have been an outstanding way to grow up, if not for her parents.

Leigh's mother had issues. Her father's issues had issues.

Leigh's father was physically and emotionally abusive, both to Leigh's mother and Leigh herself. One of Leigh's first memories is of her father beating her mother. She doesn't refer to him as father, though, or dad, or even sperm donor. The "name" she uses to refer to him is the "Psychopath." Leigh has a dark sense of humor, though she isn't kidding about this.

Her mother was married to the Psychopath twice. They married and divorced, then married and divorced again. The final split, and the last contact Leigh has ever had with him, was when she was fourteen. Though Leigh had effectively divorced from him long before fourteen, she completely disowned him then. This was sometime around when he finally put her mother in the hospital after a beating, and that was a beating so bad she had no choice but to go to the hospital. There were plenty of times she should have gone before that. It was also around the time he threw Leigh into a plate-glass door. Whether he intended it to break, and possibly kill her, she does not know. It didn't. But he still brought her to the ground and beat her with a vengeance. If there had been a relationship of any kind before that, the plate-glass door broke that. Though this is all horrifying and tragic, as abuse always is, the more complex relationship was between Leigh and her mother.

In the simplest terms, Leigh's mother had self-esteem issues. There are theories as to why, but she wasn't a terribly reflective person, and what was buried deep, and why she felt the need to project that onto Leigh, will simply never be known. Leigh's mother has passed away, and despite their confusing, damaging, and volatile past, her passing was deeply devastating for Leigh. Not surprisingly, Leigh had always dreamed her mother would someday be more of a mother, the kind of mother she imagined one could be. But her early passing made the possibility of that, or any mutual resolution, impossible.

It's not that Leigh grew up without a strong mother figure. Her grandmother, her mother's mother, was a wonderful surrogate. And though she could not undo the damage from the nuclear home, it is clear from Leigh's surprising functionality that the grandmother made a strong impact. Leigh adored her grandmother, and the feeling was mutual. Thankfully she lived down the street, as she was the only one who gave Leigh any unconditional love, not to mention meals.

Leigh's grandmother was an unusual woman by circumstance. Her life experiences were anything but usual. Leigh's grandmother was raised in the Philippines, with an American father and British mother. She bore two children during World War II, Leigh's mother and her twin brother. Three months after the babies were born, Leigh's grandmother and grandfather, the two babies, and Leigh's great-grandmother were captured and placed in a Japanese prison camp in Manila, where they all lived as prisoners of war for nearly five years. A Japanese prison camp during World War II is about as horrific as you can imagine. Although there may have been worse prison camps throughout history, and even throughout that war, this was bad enough.

There was almost no food or water in the camp for the prisoners. They had rations, but they were modest to say the least. Although there are few photographs of the Japanese camps, when Leigh's grandmother describes what it was like to have no food for years on end, she reflects on the many photographs of the Holocaust victims. Not comparing the tragedies in all respects, the people in the Japanese camps looked like those in the Nazi camps. Starving looks like starving. Needless to say, they were all very sick as well. Thankfully, MacArthur went back in during the war and freed the prisoners, or Leigh's family would all be long dead before she ever existed.

Still, recovery from five years in a prison camp is serious business. And those twin babies had spent nearly all of their first five years as prisoners of war—surrounded by starvation, sickness, violence, terror, and guarded by soldiers and guns. It would be impossible to calculate the kind of damage that would do to small children. And Leigh's mother never discussed it. Whatever devastation occurred, Leigh's mother either wasn't consciously aware of it, or was unwilling to talk about it. It would be rather absurd, however, not to assume there were consequences. The twin brother did not turn out to be a nice man. A prison camp is hardly a nurturing environment.

After the internment, it took some time for everyone to gain back their health; after all, they had been starving for a long time. Eventually, Leigh's grandmother began to put on weight and over time became quite large. Food was looked at very differently after years of not having any. Though there wasn't an excess, Leigh's grandmother ensured there was enough. She took pride in cooking and in feeding her family: Food was love, and conversely, lack of food was hate. When your captors starve you, that becomes evident. Mostly the adults returned to their hearty, natural forms.

Leigh's mother, though—whether it was because she saw her own mother get quite fat, or the social pressures from being an adolescent and teen in regular society, or some complex combination of psychological stressors that ran very deep and were never addressed—became obsessed with her weight, and in turn, her daughter's. Additionally, the Psychopath was a large man who came from a family of large people. He was a dieter. And that exacerbated the concerns her mother had about Leigh's size. Whatever the underlying causes for the paranoia, they were totally unwarranted, because Leigh was not in the slightest bit overweight, although her mother managed to make her believe she was huge—Leigh thought she was "big as a house."

Leigh's mother put her on her first diet at around age six. They would diet together. Her mother would pick whatever fad was happening at the moment and she would enroll them together. Leigh remembers weighing and measuring for Weight Watchers; they did Atkins, Beverly Hills, and all the latest and greatest. Her mom tried to get Leigh involved, on board, one of the converted. Not so much on the bandwagon, Leigh remembers her school lunches as being totally different from those of her friends, and it was humiliating. She felt there must be something terribly wrong with her that she should be treated differently. Why her? She must be bad and in need of punishment, not to mention repair. What other conclusion was there at that age? Plus her mother would tell anyone who would listen about their mother-daughter dieting, which only served to alienate and make Leigh feel alienated by others even more.

Ironically, or not, neither Leigh nor her mother were fat, or overweight, or large, or could even stand to lose a few pounds.

The problem was not in the excess tissue, but in the excess fear. Leigh's mother was certain that one additional pound would mean men wouldn't love her. She had a deep drive to be attractive to men, to feel she was attractive to men, and even more important, to be told she was attractive to men. She was nourished by compliments. She was also highly competitive with other women for men. When Leigh was fourteen, her grandmother noticed, or thought she noticed, that grown men frequently had their eye on Leigh. For reasons that were most likely generational, that pleased Leigh's grandmother. It made Leigh's mother jealous. She not only competed with other women, but she also competed with her daughter, at least in her head—Leigh had no interest in competing for men with anyone. Leigh wondered why her mother hadn't wished her fat, if fat was so unattractive and they were competing. There is no answer for that.

A longtime dieting duo, there was only one short period where meals were normal in Leigh's house. Her mother took a nine-to-five office job and Leigh was in charge of the food. She was thirteen years old. On Friday nights Leigh would plan her menu for the week. She and her mother would go shopping, and Leigh would cook for them all week long. Likely because of her grandmother's influence, Leigh enjoyed cooking and was good at it. She knew how to plan and prepare healthy, balanced meals. Proteins and vegetables, maybe a starch. Not diet food, but nutritious by most any standard. When Leigh was in charge, the house was stocked with good food, and fad diets were literally and figuratively off the table. Leigh learned not only how to prepare food, but she also learned the art of cooking—a source of pride for many, including Leigh. But for her mother, it was more a source of discomfort and worry.

A year later, Leigh's mother took care of the problem by going to work the night shift at the casino, and that ended Leigh's career as the family chef. In order to control Leigh's eating when she wasn't around, Leigh's mother stopped putting food in the house. Throughout her high school years, the kitchen cupboards were actually bare. There were times Leigh was starving. But of course not in the literal sense her family did those years before. Her grandmother would never allow that; Leigh was always fed by her with love. Though it was not lost on Leigh that the total absence of food was a peculiar way to raise a growing teenager, fat or not.

Consequently, though not surprisingly, Leigh developed an extremely distorted view of her own body. She had no sense of her actual size. Because she had been put on diets since age six, she assumed she needed them. She could fathom no logical reason to be on a diet unless there was a need to lose weight; therefore, she must need to lose weight. She always considered herself fat. Very fat. Though in objective reality, she wasn't even a little fat.

Years later, she was at her grandmother's house rifling through a drawer and came upon pictures of herself as a teenager. What she saw in those pictures was shocking and horrifying: She was perfectly normal. Not fat at all. She had no idea she hadn't been fat, being as big as a house and all. She wept over those pictures. She mourned the decades she was told she was not right, that she felt not right, that she believed so deeply that she was not right. All of those feelings were irrational regardless of her size, but then, to see evidence that blaming her size was a total distortion of reality was devastating. Even if fat was bad and somehow justified all the insecurity and dissatisfaction her mother fostered, she hadn't been fat at all. It was entirely projection. And more than that, her mother had led her to believe that because she was fat, no one would ever love her. It was a mantra she learned: "No one is ever going to love you." And then there would be another diet.

Interestingly, by the time she saw the photographs, Leigh was fat. In adulthood, she fulfilled her mother's prophecy. She ended up with the family body, and no dieting in childhood prevented it. It's hard to say how much of her weight gain was genetic, but Leigh believes a considerable amount was from a metabolism destroyed by so many years of dieting. It was not from lifelong overeating, because Leigh did not do that. While many people do end up with disordered eating of some kind because of childhood dieting, Leigh didn't.

There was one period that was an exception. The year Leigh's mother died, she fell into a deep depression. There was so much left unresolved, and it was a crushing disappointment that her mother never really became her mother. In the year after her mother's death, Leigh gained 100 pounds. She finally got big as a house, or at least fat enough that her mother would have had cause to consider her fat. The simple explanation is that Leigh filled the void of losing her mother with food. Or maybe it was some kind of tribute, or revenge. It certainly was poetic justice, in the darkest of ways. She lost some of the weight when the depression lifted, but not all of it. Undramatically, though, that was the extent of Leigh's foray into anything that could be called disordered eating.

It is actually fairly unusual that all of her childhood dieting did not lead to some kind of food conflict. Perhaps it was her grandmother who saved her from that fate. Leigh felt that her mother's love was conditional on some abstract idea of what her body must be but wasn't. Her grandmother put no conditions on her love. Additionally, Leigh's grandmother was big, and Leigh was able to love her more than anyone. Proof positive that fat and love are not mutually exclusive.

Leigh did live up to her mother's fears in a sense. She did become a fat woman. Ironically, one of the reasons she probably put on weight was that at age fifteen she stopped playing sports. Right before Leigh started high school, her grandmother, who despite her love was from a different time and place, suggested that only "certain types of girls play sports beyond her age." Leigh actually was a certain type of girl, but she was also the type of girl who wanted to please her grandmother. So she quit sports. Of course, to add irony to absurdity, being a certain type of girl, Leigh would have been no competition for men at any weight. Also, sports don't turn women into lesbians, but logic has no bearing on that kind of thinking.

Logic was something Leigh had to learn on her own, and she seemed to intuit well, for better or worse. Leigh was correct in her assessment when she was a child: You don't diet unless there is something wrong with you—that is to say you diet when you are overweight and believe being overweight is wrong. Additionally, you must believe that your weight is something you can control, and if you don't, there is also something wrong with you. That is the message Leigh learned from her mother. Her mother truly believed it. What logical reason was there for Leigh to disagree? Especially when she was as big as a house.

9

PUNISHABLE BY DEATH

illy lived in a town so small you could practically fit it in the palm of your hand. There wasn't much to do there but believe what you are told, and act accordingly. When Lilly's father left, he did so with no uncertain terms and very specific instructions for her mother: "If she turns out fat like you, I will find you and kill you." He was using his go-to weapon of choice, the one he knew would hurt Lilly's mother the most. She had always been insecure about her body. By throwing in a threat about the kid, he added a grenade to his usual arsenal. It was all hyperbole; he wasn't going to kill anyone. That doesn't mean he didn't cause casualties.

That pretty much set the tone for the rest of Lilly's childhood. From then on it was Lilly and her mother against the world—partners in crime. But they were unwitting criminals. The crime was fat, punishable by death. They did everything they could to go straight. So they dieted. It seemed their entire little town was guilty—at least their women. Population 101, all of the townswomen joined forces. As a community, they banded together to form a diet posse. They became a gang of dieters. Weight-loss marauders.

In other words, after Lilly and her mother had dealt with this man leaving, and his parting words, the town formed a diet club. And Lilly and her mother joined. Lilly was particularly successful. At one point she received an award for losing the most weight of the entire group, in essence the entire town. It might as well have been the entire planet. It was quite an honor, and a reinforcement.

The group didn't last long, however. Eventually the women began gaining back what they had lost. They felt the group was ailing, so they put it out of its misery. Or perhaps it died of natural causes. In any event, some women went off on their own to look for other diet plans and some got sick and tired of the entire thing and just let themselves be fat. The latter was not an option for Lilly and her mother, so they moved on to their next dieting stop.

Lilly was eight when her parents split and this process first began. Her mother never remarried and Lilly had no father figure to speak of, which only strengthened the notion of Lilly and her mother against the world. While all the women in her mom's family looked alike—they were fat—Lilly's dad's mother may have been fat too. There was something about his disdain for fat women that seemed tied to his mother. But Lilly can't be sure. She never got to know them and never wanted to. Lilly had a sense of protectiveness for her mother that precluded any desire to interact with her father's people, and she has had no contact with him since she was sixteen. Bluster or not, his attitude and words greatly shaped Lilly's life. At least in part because of his hostility toward fat women, Lilly became one, like her mother. His threat didn't make that happen, but it certainly influenced a chain of events.

Actually, Lilly didn't grow up to be fat like her mother. Lilly grew up to be much fatter. She says she can trace different fat parts of herself to the fat parts of her mother's family. She is a conglomeration of all the fat. Her mother was never all that fat, but nonetheless always felt she was, and therefore unattractive. Her mom was maybe, at most, a size 16. She was also massively strong, probably the strongest woman Lilly has ever met in her life.

Lilly's mother grew up on a farm; she was a dairy farmer and a lumberjack. Lumberjacks are strong. She was relatively large compared to many of the girls she grew up with and had been teased for it. She dieted constantly and had for years, except when she was depressed. She was prone to depression and when she was depressed she didn't need to diet because she didn't eat at all.

At any rate, the women on Lilly's mother's side were large. Hardworking, and large. They were poor, and Lilly grew up poor as well. But unlike most of them, Lilly was bookish. Lilly is very smart. Between being fat and smart, Lilly was also teased, and had few friends. She spent a great deal of time reading her days away. Though her mother didn't understand what she was reading, or why she was reading it, she realized reading was a good thing, important, and should be encouraged. Lilly's mother always made sure Lilly had books.

It actually wasn't until Lilly was about eleven when her mother began bringing up the topic of her weight. As many girls do, she began to put on a little when she started to hit puberty. Lilly was very active in sports, and her mother used that as a "motivational tool." She told Lilly that if she didn't lose weight they would be forced to throw her off the volleyball team because they wouldn't have a uniform to fit her. Lilly didn't exactly buy that, she realized uniforms probably came in her size, but it still managed to prompt her first diet. That summer, Lilly lived with her aunt to help babysit the children. Everyone there dieted together.

Her first diet with her mother as partner was when she was about thirteen and just entering junior high. They had a food plan book with serving exchanges used by diabetics: One slice of bread is the same as six crackers—and so forth. They followed it religiously. They then took a trip to Nutrisystem, which many seem to worship. After doing the calculations, Lilly and her mom determined it would cost $22.44 for each pound lost, if everything went perfectly. Too rich for their blood. At age fourteen they finally started TOPS (Take Off Pounds Sensibly), and so did much of the town. TOPS wasn't particularly effective at taking off pounds, nor was it particularly sensible. But they had good advertising.

There was a weekly meeting and weigh-in. Lilly won that award for losing the most weight. She had lost the most weight in her group, but she also, apparently, lost the most weight in the state. It's not entirely clear how the state determined that, but they awarded her for it. When she inevitably gained the weight back in college, she was forced to return her sash and crown.

Lilly and her mother did not initially argue about weight— Lilly agreed with her mother that she needed to lose it. But as she matured, so did her ideas about dieting; their fighting began when Lilly was seventeen and continued until she turned thirty. Prior to arguing about weight, their main subject of dispute was religion. Lilly's mother was a staunch Catholic and Lilly, during what might be considered her budding rebellion, "just didn't feel it." Partly, the influence was all those books she had been reading. Some were on feminism, and over time she became a card-carrying member. As Lilly began to conceive of the world from a feminist perspective, her point of view began to diverge from her mother's. It began as disagreement about Catholicism; eventually they crossed on broader issues, including weight.

It's not like Lilly had been raised on fast-food, or even processed diet foods. Despite assumptions many make about fat people, the meals Lilly's mother prepared would be considered nearly ideal. They ate vegetables from their garden. They raised chickens and rabbits as livestock. Lilly's mother baked all her own bread. In fact, her mom made everything they ate, and virtually all the ingredients came from the backyard. There weren't even desserts; neither Lilly nor her mother had much of a sweet tooth. Had they simply eaten instead of dieted, perhaps things would have turned out differently.

About ten years ago, Lilly's mother was diagnosed with diabetes, which runs in the family. At that point, Lilly's mother sort of mutated from being a chronic dieter to being compulsive with food. It became a daily obsession that nearly dominates her life. She has developed virtually uncontrollable urges to eat things she had never craved before, like packaged dinner rolls, Wonder Bread, and cake. Why, exactly, is speculation. It is not speculation, however, that Lilly cut off all conversation with her mother about dieting and weight.

It's not that Lilly found peace with her size. But the topic had become too painful, even if her mother was motivated by love and concern. They still both believed Lilly's life would be happier, and she would be healthier, if she were thinner. To that end, Lilly took a drastic and surprising step. Despite her newly enlightened beliefs about feminism, culture, and weight, the drive to be thin was too powerful, as was the fear about continuing to be fat. Lilly had begun searching for professional jobs. She was certain that any employer would view her size as a deficit— of willpower, determination, and even character. Lilly couldn't imagine being hired, and even if she could, she was certain she would be forced through humiliating extra interviews, that proving her worth would be exceptionally difficult and require extraordinary circumstances.

So Lilly decided to, as some are wont to say, "finally take care of the problem." Lilly prepared for weight-loss surgery. This— making it impossible for her to be the glutton fat people are accused of being—was the one thing the doctors believed could rid her of her massive burden. Prior to this time, she had been dieting and exercising strenuously, and was still gaining weight. She underwent six months of tests. Lilly had psychological tests, metabolic tests, blood tests, was tested for sleep apnea, and to top it off, she kept food diaries. In conclusion, all of the medical professionals determined that her metabolism didn't work right, and the fix was surgery on her stomach.

Lilly spoke with her mother about the plan, expecting her to be thrilled at this life-altering step. Her mother wasn't unhappy, but she wasn't thrilled. She was surprisingly circumspect. Perhaps because she was an old-school dieter, this didn't sit well with her. Some people think it's the "easy way out." Perhaps she was jealous. Or maybe she was simply afraid for her daughter. But she wasn't against it. They hadn't talked about weight in many years—Lilly wouldn't allow it, and her mother only wanted for her daughter to find happiness and success. Weight-loss surgery could be the golden ticket.

Lilly had a Roux-en-Y gastric bypass, then and now considered one of the safest and most effective weight-loss surgeries, and one still commonly performed today. With the Roux-en-Y, a small stomach pouch is created with a stapler device, and connected to the farthest part of the small intestine. The upper part of the small intestine is then reattached in a Y-shaped configuration. Lilly was still relatively young when she had her surgery, and in an effort to prevent malabsorption, a frequent and serious consequence of weight-loss surgery, the doctors made her pouch larger than they normally do. They realized she needed her stomach to continue working for a long time.

That was the plan, at any rate.

Lilly had complications almost immediately. At first they were psychological. Although Lilly had excellent pre-op care (which some people don't), she wasn't as prepared as she had imagined. She was unable to accept the idea that she had to mutilate her body to become normal. Lilly did lose 136 pounds in four months—which, depending on your perspective, is great, or horrifying. But then the weight loss stopped, and Lilly became suicidally depressed. There was no long-term follow-up mental health care at the weight-loss center, so she found a psychologist who had expertise in body dysmorphia and eating disorders. Now, after the surgery and losing all that weight, Lilly developed an eating disorder. She stopped eating altogether; she would go for days without eating anything, and since she felt no hunger, there was no drive to eat. Even so, she stopped losing, and actually started gaining, which somehow others perceived as her fault.

That is when the "real" complications started. She became tired. Beyond tired. She developed a severe B12 deficiency, which requires injections for the rest of her life. And then there was the pain— crouched-on-the-floor-in-a-ball pain. She had a kidney stone so big it took three surgeries over two and a half weeks to remove. And then another one. One every month. Every month, to this day. Later the anemia was diagnosed, three types, causing neurological brain and kidney damage. The cause: malabsorption of nutrients. So much for the special measures taken by the docs to make sure her stomach worked. The long shot, Lilly will be sick and need continual medical care for the rest of her life, which they estimate will be ten to fifteen years shorter than if she had never had the surgery, and had just stayed fat. She's fat again, by the way. She gained back at least half of what she had lost.

Lilly and her mother no longer talk about weight loss at all. What is there to say, really?

Regardless of how it turned out, Lilly believes everything her mother did was out of love. She was concerned about Lilly's health and also her social life. She had been raised to believe fat girls never find husbands, have families, get good jobs, or feel loved. Lilly's mother recognized the prejudice against fat people, and she didn't want that for her daughter. And frankly, Lilly's mother wasn't entirely wrong. Prejudice is very real. But when it comes to fat children, there are the wrong ways to handle helping, and very few other options—whatever those other options may be, Lilly's mother had never been schooled.

During one epic fight, Lilly's mother said, "You have such a pretty face, if only you . . ." Lilly says, "I remember yelling at her, 'What you're telling me is that I'm ugly and I'm also a failure because I'm not living up to what you think I should be.' It was the first time she ever got the idea that even if she was speaking out of concern, her language had an effect, and it was painful." After the surgery, and after gaining much of the weight back, Lilly saw an advertisement for a clinical study related to weight loss. She called and explained to them about the gastric bypass and her circumstances. Their response: "We're sorry you didn't have success with the surgery; it's a shame." "I had to rip my guts apart to become what was considered normal, and I never got close to normal. They felt that was a shame, my lack of success. I lost 100 pounds and I still wasn't successful."

Language has an effect. Though Lilly felt her mother was loving in many ways, and for a good deal of her life believed her mother was right in caring about her weight, it wasn't harmless caring.

That was all that I ever heard, I mean the doctors talked about it, the PE teachers talked about it, people on television talked about it, magazines talked about it. It was all about how you have to lose weight, you have to change your diet. I remember when the food pyramid changed and carbohydrates became good, but they never told us white pasta was not so good. My relationship with my mother and myself with regards to weight started to change as I became a feminist. I started to think about my own life and my mother's life, and I saw how much of that diet focus was about the controlling of women's bodies. Until after I had my gastric bypass surgery I still really believed that losing weight was the right thing to do. It wasn't until afterwards when I started getting really sick, and had to start trying to find ways to come to grips with it, rebuild my life, think about my decisions in a new way—a critical way— that I really looked at the messages I had been getting, that I had been listening to my whole life. I realized it didn't work for me, there's something not right. It probably was a good two or three years after my surgery that I got to a point where I could say the message that weight and health are automatically connected is not necessarily right. I still struggle with this today; I probably will my entire life.

Eventually Lilly went on to study weight, study children and weight. She became a social scientist, she studied education— what and how children learn. Of course she was interested in herself as well—what she'd learned and how she'd learned it all. A natural outgrowth, she studied girls, and their relationships with their mothers. She came across an article—the research suggested that girls who were overweight or obese were the least likely to go on to college, and if they did, they were the least likely to graduate. Lilly had finished college; in fact she was in graduate school. She was getting a PhD. How did that connect with what she had learned, and her mother?

What she learned from the girls she studied, girls who were over-weight or obese, was that they felt they had no one to look up to, and no one to talk to. They felt that heavier people were not visible as positive role models, so they had no image of success to imagine for themselves. She also learned from the girls she studied that they wanted to talk about their families. They wanted to talk about how the messages they got at home impacted them. They didn't want to lament abuse, per se—in fact many said they had very caring families. But caring or not, the conversations about weight and weight loss were so frequent, so pervasive, that the family became a hostile environment. Many would stop interacting with their families altogether. But even when they did, those messages had already impacted their sense of themselves. The girls didn't feel capable. Not capable of learning. They felt it didn't matter how well they did in school. It didn't matter if they got pregnant young and out of wedlock. Losing weight was all that mattered, and when they couldn't lose weight they were failures. In fact, if you were fat, nothing really mattered. And they were fat, so they didn't matter.

Lilly might have said the same thing about her family—her mother and herself—when she was young. She has clearer perspective now. But to gain that perspective, she had life experiences no caring family would wish upon a daughter. Lilly is in a good place now, considering. She manages her chronic health problems. She got a job. She found a husband. She has great insight into her life that she might not have had otherwise. She says she doesn't resent the journey because it brought her to a good place. Still, if she could have reached that place without so many twists and turns, she would have taken that road instead.

There can be such a fine line between help and harm. That line is so thin, so tenuous, it is often hard to recognize. And children are eminently fragile. The best intentions sometimes have the worst consequences. There is more than one kind of death. One can experience death of hope, and dreams, of future, and worth, of place in the world, and sense of self. All of that can happen when that fine line is crossed, and then, fat is punishable by death.

10

FAT AND HAPPY

Both of Eric's parents were raised during the Depression. Despite challenging times, they were encouraged to be smart and take those smarts far. Their parents' generation were nobody's fool. Eric's father went to medical school via the army and became a psychiatrist. His mother graduated high school at sixteen, got a scholarship to college, and became a doctor in a hospital. Though the household Eric grew up in was middle class by any standards, there was more of a working-class vibe about the home.

> I was raised in a 90 percent working-class neighborhood. My parents had money but they lived several notches below. I wasn't raised with a silver spoon like other doctors' kids. My dad said money is for rainy days, education, and for taking trips. "Just because I've got money doesn't mean I've got money to waste." So I couldn't have fashionable clothes with labels and cars.

There were no fancy cars or ostentatious trinkets, but there was food. Always plenty of food. That was carried over from the Depression-era days, where hunger was always staring them square in the face, and if there was opportunity for food, it was gotten, and eaten. It was to some degree a sign of success, to have ample if not abundant nourishment, but more so it was merely a reaction to the past. You simply never know what is around the next corner. In addition to that dynamic, Eric and his family are black, and it wasn't so many generations ago that having a bountiful table was completely unknown.

Though Eric was raised in the East, his family lineage, at least for several generations back, was Southern. So that also had an impact. Culturally, a plentiful table was encouraged and the bounty should include all kinds, if not every kind, of Southern delight. Multiple meats with eggs, and pancakes, and grits, was not uncommon on the breakfast table, and the entire family was encouraged to enjoy. Food felt good, physically, emotionally, as a foundation for bonding, to demonstrate an environment of safety and comfort, and as a cover for issues people preferred to evade.

So, everyone in Eric's family was pretty fat. Mom and Dad, his kid brother who is five years younger, and Eric himself. Whether that was an issue sort of depended on the day. Sometimes his dad would get angry, particularly at Eric's younger brother, who was the fatter of the two. For no reason apparent to Eric, out of the blue his father would complain, especially to his brother, "You're too fat; you enjoy your food too much." They all enjoyed their food, that was really the point, and in no uncertain terms. But the mood would strike him, and Dad got pissed. At one point, Eric's brother was brought to a pediatrician, a family friend from college, who told the eight-year-old boy that if he didn't lose weight he would get really fat, have a heart attack, and die. Eric's brother was quite traumatized by that, which didn't change the dynamic at home. But it stuck with the kid, and not for the better.

Outside the house, both Eric and his brother were teased. It wasn't a tragic amount of teasing, but it's not like Eric has forgotten about it, either. They also got teased for being smart kids. Today, perhaps they would be considered nerds, which in some circles is cool, but in the '60s in their neighborhood, a brainiac had no redeeming value to his peers. Luckily for Eric, he could throw a mean one-liner, as well as a football. He became obsessed with football at around nine and that was his saving grace. He played. It was just pickup games, but tackle, so Eric's size was to his advantage, even if his running was a little slow. Plus, he knew everything about the pros, the player and their stats. In that regard, being a brainiac was more of a crutch.

Eric first attempted to slim down when he started to like girls. In the sixth grade, just when he was hitting puberty, one mean girl told him he was fat, and that his hair was too nappy and he couldn't dress. That was her opinion, and although Eric believed her, he wasn't all that fat. Hair and clothes, that's certainly subjective. But he decided then if he was fat, with bad hair and ugly clothes, he had better be funny and cool. He also started to be conscious of what he ate—for instance, he would drain the oil from his tuna fish. He believes now that his perception of himself as fat worked to his advantage. It motivated him. And it was true he didn't have "good hair," wavy like Billy Dee Williams's character in the *Star Wars* movie. But that look didn't last forever. Once "black awareness" became popular, so did nappy hair. Eric also became a creative dresser. He decided to be ahead of the pack. A growth spurt and some John Lennon glasses helped, as did the time he was walking with his mom and she noticed a girl looking at him and smiling. He thought his mom was teasing. He carried that fat kid thing with him still, but the times they were a-changing.

Despite the fact that Eric started making attempts to lose weight at around age twelve, and that at the time he was five feet eight inches tall and 120 pounds, he had carried the burden of being a fat kid for years. Still, by college, Eric was trading on his great personality. He couldn't imagine women would find him attractive for any other reason. There was a woman in college who had the tallest Afro in school, was a dead ringer for Pam Grier—but despite the fact that the rumor mill claimed she had the hots for him, there was no way that Eric could believe it. It all started with a few teasing incidents, and that girl in the sixth grade who read him the riot act, and the perception of others became reality.

He would think about the kid he had been, the one in the middle-class home with food being served like it was a generation before in the poverty-stricken Deep South. Never a salad or a

piece of fresh fruit. Eric would come home from school and ritu-
alistically make himself two peanut butter and jelly sandwiches,
sometimes three, watch cartoons, and have another snack before
dinner. And although his brother got grief for being tubby, that
didn't change the meal plan, or the fact that his parents, fat themselves, were always snacking too. It was a stress reliever, and a
memory reliever. There was plenty of talk about cleaning your
plate because in the 1930s, they barely had meat. Forty years ago,
the family was poor and suffering, and they were still making up
for it. It was their history and their heritage.

Eric and his brother laugh about it now, but the cognitive dissonance between being berated for being fat, then told to clean
your plate to avoid starvation, was not lost on the boys. It's true
that Eric's brother was the heavier of the two, but that doesn't
quite account for the fact that it was really only he who was singled out. Everyone was fat, at least at one point or another. But
this kid was a scapegoat for something. He was a super sweet boy,
the kind who would never fight back. That might have been part
of it. Eric's dad was under a lot of stress as well—just because
life is stressful, but also because he had a lot to live up to as a
first-generation black man of the middle-class, and doctor.

His own father was a preacher, and an alcoholic. His father,
Eric's great-grandfather, was a freed slave. The grandfather had
been raised with corporal punishment, which is a more polite way
to say brutal whippings. Eric's father was also subject to the belt.
He would be required to bring that belt into the bath with him so
his father (Eric's granddad) could take care of business. Granddad,
as stated, was the son of a freed man, and as such he had the opportunity to earn a master's in divinity. Educated and proud, he was
frustrated with life in the '20s, '30s, and '40s, forced to do odd jobs
despite his credentials and abilities. He turned to drink, and continued the pattern of harsh punishment when the stress and strain became too much. Each succeeding generation of men went lighter on
the physical reprimands, and by the time Eric and his brother came
around, the tactics were all psychological, but not without impact.

Perhaps Eric's father was conflicted about his son's weight because, like generations before him, he had grown up with conflict around food. The granddad, being a man of the cloth, was responsible for serving itinerant preachers who would come for Sunday supper—Sunday being the one day of the week the family would eat meat. Many Sundays there would be some random preacher sitting at the family table, eating the lion's share of the pork chops. And leaving Eric's father without. So, yes, there was a contradiction in encouraging his sons to eat to their hearts' content, and then displaying annoyance that they got fat for the love of food. But his ability to provide and keep his sons well fed was a source of great pride, though not one that he had any experience or training moderating. He loved his sons more than anything and at one point, as a psychiatrist, actually analyzed himself for this behavior. He realized he wished he had been kinder. Eric learned this much later, but he did notice that when he was around twelve or thirteen his father seemed to change. He became more mellow. There was still the occasional outburst, but mostly he'd happily say, "Kids, eat up, it's a great pot roast," and there would be storytelling and laughter around the table.

When Eric was ten, his mother was diagnosed with a disease similar to lupus. It's one of those diseases that affect black women more frequently than white, a disease in which the immune system attacks the connective tissue. It was a slow degenerative disease, and that impacted the entire family. They could never be certain when to expect a flare-up. Shortly after diagnosis, she began to miss days working as a doctor and in turn spent those days sick as a patient. When Eric was fifteen and his little brother was ten, their mother had a heart attack and died. Though Eric was devastated, of course, both his brother and father were more prone to anxiety. Food helped them cope, and fat ran in the family.

On both sides, the relatives were bigger, the aunts and uncles and cousins. Eric would visit, and for him, it would be like a festival of food, but for them, that was everyday life. Culturally, fat and happy was big in the black community, far more so than following fashion trends, or being paranoid about health. Perhaps because Eric's parents were both doctors, it wasn't quite as easy for them to totally disregard the issues of weight and illness, whether real or imagined. Still, all that really amounted to was that Eric's family felt bad about themselves in a way the relatives didn't.

Eric's cousins were much fatter than he or his brother, yet they had none of the emotional strain. They never felt fat and ugly. They were sassy with women, even as boys. At around fourteen, tall for their age, they would sneak into bars, and the cousins would think nothing of going right up to a woman: "Hey, foxy mama, what's up?" That was never Eric's scene. It was so inconceivable, really, that Eric and his brother would joke that their cousins were too dumb to realize they were fat and ugly and couldn't get women. But in fact, they weren't dumb at all; they both grew up to be very successful professionals, with hot women to boot.

It was only upon adult reflection that Eric realized the importance of perception. "They made me realize how much is in your own mind. I still deal with that myself; here I am, I've been married and divorced and I've had many girlfriends, and I still tell myself if I just lose 30 pounds, I will be able to talk to a woman. But these guys have had hot babes all their lives. They didn't think like me." Not that the cousins were immune from many of the usual indignities fat people suffer. One cousin's doctor told him his heart was filled with mashed potatoes. That, it is safe to assume, is a medical impossibility. And Eric's brother never recovered from the shame he felt about being fat, and he never had success with women, which Eric concludes is mostly because of his head, not his gut.

Eric's weight fluctuated as a boy, as it did when he got older. At one point, he weighed in at about 300 pounds. There is a genetic component in that family; it's not all about Southern cooking. In fact, at various times in Eric's life, he was a vegetarian. True, health wasn't his primary motivator—the impetus for these periods was usually a vegetarian woman, and when the woman went away, the meat and potatoes came back. But to be fair, food was not the single determinant of Eric's weight, one way or another. And it wasn't inactivity; Eric was always active. But despite his genetic makeup, and whatever other factors came into play, it was Eric's perception that food was the primary culprit of any excess weight. This was reinforced with information from doctors, such as his cousin's heart was filled with mashed potatoes. Perception.

Eric became interested in whole foods and what is now the farm-to-table movement much earlier than most. Ironically, it came out of his love for chocolate. When Eric was twelve, his father won an award and they took a trip to San Francisco, where they visited Ghirardelli Square. The place where chocolate is made. A factory filled with vats of chocolate is a magical land for a twelve-year-old, and Eric just knew he must live there some day. To make it all the more glamorous, they dined in a restaurant that allowed you to pick your own slice of meat—the cut and the size. Prior to this, Eric didn't have much of an understanding of where food came from, beyond the market. In this city, they too had food co-ops, with fresh vegetables direct from the farmers, and chickens that had not been processed in a factory. This being the early 1960s, it was only the beginning of prepackaged consumables, but the place in which Eric lived was strictly urban. He had been raised to love food, and here they understood food.

Eric did, in fact, end up living in that special place at one point. Despite the chocolate, he became so thin from the healthy eating, constant walking, and manual labor, that upon returning home, his family was convinced he was using heroin. Like so many, the story of Eric's weight loss, and gain, is lengthy. And frankly, it's not all that interesting, unless you like to hear tales of beer and pizza, followed by new trainers at the gym. Or brown rice and broccoli, followed by breakfasts of brandy Alexanders with raw egg and heavy cream. Or perhaps good marriages with fresh green salads, followed by divorces and takeout Chinese. Life has its ups and downs.

After Eric's mother passed, his father married a woman with a keen interest in t'ai chi and fad foods. When fat was the popular enemy, they ate loads of pasta. When carbs were evil, meat ruled. This woman was also white and Jewish, and had a different cultural attitude toward food than the one with whom Eric was raised. At one point Eric become prediabetic and his doctor told him if he got full-blown diabetes, he would go blind, have his feet amputated from gangrene, develop liver and kidney disease, and die slowly, in agony. So for various reasons, sometimes Eric was fatter, and sometimes he was not.

As so many who have struggled with weight do, Eric often contemplates how much of all this is genetic and beyond his control, and how much is his own damn fault. There is no question having ample food available at all times was a source of pleasure with his family. "That was reinforced by both my parents: "'We have plenty of food.' My dad would tell us, 'When your mother and I were kids, it was government cheese and canned vegetables, and now we can eat up. Pass the potatoes and help yourself.' He would invite friends for big meals, boasting how 'We have plenty of food.' It was a great source of pride." But pride in bountiful food is not unique to Eric's family. Such abundance brings satisfaction all over the planet and has been for as long as there was also starvation. This is often the case, even for those who don't have a history with government cheese and canned vegetables.

> I've got friends my age, one who is Chinese American, he's 59, and we saw some pictures of ourselves in 1988 and he looks exactly the same. He hasn't gained a bit of weight and he can eat way more than me. If I really chow down, like, to be in a food coma, he can keep going past that point. I do think it's both what you eat and genetics. People in my family, unless they really watch their weight, they end up fat and with diseases. But friends of mine eat what they want and plenty of it, don't exercise, and are still skinny. They just have that kind of metabolism.

Unlike what might be the case today, Eric's parents, the doctors, did not feel a particular pressure to assure the healthiest eating. That may have been in part because of their medical specialties, his dad being a psychiatrist and his mom working mostly with geriatric patients in acute care. Now, doctors perhaps feel more shame if they are fat and perceived as unhealthy. Additionally, at least then, there was a cultural difference, being black, and also living and working with the poor. Some might argue that hasn't entirely changed today, and both certain research and a great amount of gossip suggests that the African American and poor cultures are more tolerant of a large stature, and perhaps less rigorous about health. This doesn't entirely explain why fat was only a fleeting concern. Eric's father had a variety of patients, and an extremely successful practice. He was well regarded in his city, one that certainly had its share of competent doctors. And Eric's mother died fairly young, being followed by a stepmother who was in fact "up to date" on the latest in healthy eating, if fad eating is considered healthy.

Whether or not it is any different in most families, Eric believed they had a long history of "eating the blues away." Also, eating for celebration. "Things are great, who wants ice cream?" "Things are lousy, who wants ice cream?" It was practically a family motto. Although things were sometimes great, there was a fair amount of lousy. And there was a lot of eating during the six years Eric's mother was sick. But even before that strain, Eric's mother had a good deal to eat over. Her father was what they politely called a "colorful character." As the story goes, he once lost an eye attempting to molest a woman factory worker, when she jabbed him in the socket with a hot rivet. He managed to steal from the New Jersey mob, then proceeded to jump a freight train and become a hobo. His wife—upon finding a picture of a pregnant woman in his wallet he claimed was a cousin—beat him with a pan. Stories like these are what Eric's dad called the family ghosts, and there were all sorts. There were also anxieties, from situations real and imagined, as a result of living through the

Great Depression, and additionally being poor and black. "We eat a lot to deal with that." And understandably so. The second wife tried to curb that response in Eric's father; in fact, she went to great lengths at times.

> My father used to sneak downstairs to where my stepmother would keep cakes and pies in the freezer for parties and Christmas. In the middle of the night he would secretly, or so he thought, cut through the frozen cake, eat the middle, and return the rest of the evidence to be found later. To stop him, she found a long chain, which she wrapped all around the freezer, then secured with a giant padlock. "We're not going to have you die because you're sawing through frozen cake." She would also monitor his car, searching for Hostess wrappers, which she would find frequently. He died at seventy-six, and I do think her tactics added a good ten to fifteen years onto his life.

Whether she fostered a longer life, no one really knows. But Eric grew up believing that was the case.

With all his contemplating, ruminating, and fretting, there is a part of Eric that considers the whole weight thing blown out of proportion. It depends on when and why the issue comes up.

> We all carry our weight so well people don't notice it that much. I don't notice it. It's like I swell up slowly, the arms get bigger, the chest, the thighs, the neck, the face, and then all of a sudden I realize, "Oh my God, I really am fat." We are also blessed with really strong bodies. It's a blessing and a curse because all of a sudden I'm adding up all this weight—and I'm strong so I can carry it around. It's not like I'm some guy who needs a cane or a walker because my legs are giving out.

Nonetheless, to this day Eric continues to attempt to lose weight, or maintain weight loss, depending what phase he is in. These days, Eric visits a naturopath to aid in the process. He does cleansing fasts. Currently, if he loses another 30 pounds he will weigh what he weighed in 1987, and that idea pleases him a great deal.

> We all grow old and we're all going to die one way or another, but I'm not going to help myself. I've had plenty of booze and pasta and spaghetti sauce. It's a daily struggle. The hardest thing for me is beer. I love beer. I wouldn't think I was drinking that much beer, but I was having two to five beers a day, just in the natural course of things. By just cutting beer I went down 10 pounds in 2 weeks. And I drank a lot of juice, which is pure sugar. I'm slowly training myself how to eat and drink better. Now I'll have like two tablespoons of rice instead of a plateful. Or four or five French fries with a burger. Just a few tastes so good. I used to eat fifty French fries and not even think about it. Once a month I have pad Thai noodles and I want to cry it tastes so good, but that's all I need. I'm trying to train myself to eat healthy and boring foods.

And there is certainly nothing wrong with training oneself to eat healthy (albeit boring) foods. It's just that this is not Eric's first go-round. He's been a vegetarian, and then he hasn't. He's been athletic, and then he hasn't. He's gone for the brown rice and broccoli, and then back to pizza and beer. Maybe it's all about moderation, and maybe moderation can be learned. It didn't work for anyone else in Eric's family, unless you count a padlocked freezer as a successful lesson plan. But despite his father telling him—on some days—that the family should be fat and happy, Eric has never liked being fat—it never made him happy. His cousins were fat and happy, but they weren't given all those conflicting messages. Being fat and happy, it seems, takes a great deal of training as well, and there are far fewer teachers of that.

11

WALKING THE GAUNTLET

The neighborhood called Eleanor Bruno's family the "Fat Brunos," because they were all fat, and, well, because the neighborhood was a tad sadistic. It is a fact that Eleanor, or Ellie, and her entire family were fat. Both her parents were fat, and she and her three siblings were fat. Though they certainly were not the only fat people in the neighborhood, they were the only entire fat family. There was a family one neighborhood over who were also all fat, and chances are they had a nickname too, but Ellie kept her distance from this family. Not out of contempt—she felt deeply for them—but out of pure self-preservation. Being associated with one fat family was more than enough for anyone in that town to cope with. Sadistic tendencies had no neighborhood boundaries, and she suspected they were cumulative, if not exponential.

Ellie says that by today's standards her parents weren't really all that fat; in fact, they were what we might now call Average Americans. But people in the 1970s were less fat, and Ellie's perception of how fat people used to be, and how badly they were treated relative to today, was not completely objective. But being a member of the Fat Brunos was enough to distort anyone's perceptions, especially that of a little kid who had no other perspective to compare. And besides, Average Americans are called fat all the time.

What was true was that her parents were each the heaviest members of their respective families, and that didn't help matters of perception. Her father was particularly stigmatized within his own family, and then, as well as now, had fixations with food and weight, which he projected liberally on his own fat children.

Ellie's mother was not so afflicted, primarily because her own mother, Ellie's maternal grandmother, made sure of it. When Ellie's mom was a little girl, her mother noticed that the child had not yet dropped her "baby fat" by the time it was expected to be dropped. Also, she and her elder sister, eighteen months her senior, were the same size. Puzzlingly, Ellie's mom was relatively bigger for her age despite eating the same food, doing the same amount of exercise, and essentially spending every waking and sleeping moment with her sibling. Ellie's grandmother's motherly instinct told her something was not right. So Ellie's grandmother carted her daughter off to a specialist who ran tests, which would most typically reveal that the child was simply a lazy glutton.

Surprisingly, the results revealed something else—that Ellie's mom had a slow thyroid and metabolism. The specialist informed her, "This is just the way she is; it's not her fault and you should not blame her for it. There is no point in putting her on a diet. She is otherwise healthy and we are all different." You mean her fat is not a result of bad character or moral decrepitude? That was daresay even more astounding in the 1950s than it would be today, as then everyone was blamed for their own perceived shortcomings. Actually that's about the same as today. However, Ellie's grandmother took the diagnosis quite seriously—a fancy learned doctor came to such a conclusion. It was a great relief for a mother to find out they weren't complicit in their child's abnormality. Consequently, Ellie's mom was never put on a diet, not made to feel ashamed, and simply grew up to be fatter than her sister—and then proceeded to have fat children herself.

Of course that didn't stop other people from casting blame and insults; they hadn't been privy to the doctor's conclusions, and probably wouldn't have believed them anyway because, well, people can be like that.

Ellie was not only the eldest of four children each six years apart; she was also the fattest. Between them, there were four young children and two young parents. No one was prepared. To add to the mix, Ellie's father was not the most consistent bread-winner and there was always a fear there might not be enough bread, as well as the accompanying meal. There was, but a sense of anxiety around food was pervasive in the house, both because of potential scarcity and because by looking at their bellies some mistakenly assumed there was an ill-consumed abundance. Food, though, was an important cultural aspect of family life. Italian on the father's side and Polish on the mother's, celebratory feast-ing was done as often as there was cause to celebrate. Ellie's grandmother on her father's side, the Italian side, was particu-larly fond of preparing massive family feasts and encouraging everyone to "eat up, eat up." Not part of the cliché of the Italian grandmother was the passive-aggressive play that was a floor-show with the meal.

This grandmother was quite slender, in fact the most slender of the family, and though she liked to cook, it appeared she liked to serve up guilt just as much. After each hearty meal, when people's pants were unbuttoned and the eating up turned to satiety, the grandmother would feed her ego by running her hands down her sides and note how slender she managed to remain—unlike the rest of them. She would point out her still willowy figure and how she exercised to maintain it, with the caveat that before bearing her son, Ellie's father, she was even more glorious, and in fact had been ruined by the pregnancy.

She then proceeded to berate others for their undisciplined heftiness. Ellie's mother learned to loathe the words "eat up," as she knew what was next on the menu. At the time Ellie didn't yet know what being fat meant, or that she resembled that remark. But as soon as she was old enough to understand, her grand-mother directed her projection and condemnation where she believed it was deserved. Up until that point, Ellie spent a good deal of time with her grandmother on weekends. But when Ellie became a target, her mother swiftly put an end to it by limiting access. Ellie's mother never criticized her for her weight. Never mentioned diets. She did what she could, little as that might have been, to protect Ellie from insult—just as her own mother had done for her.

While Ellie's mother tried her very best to protect her from abuse for being fat, she was not terribly successful, not at the dinner table, and particularly not out in the world. And despite her best attempts at protection, she didn't always succeed with her own messages. When Ellie was eleven, her mother witnessed her daughter being ridiculed at the supermarket. Ellie was off running after a sibling as her mother was on the checkout line, and two of the checkout girls caught a glimpse of each other, rolled their eyes, and said something about Ellie's fat ass. The very next day Ellie's mother put her in a girdle. It was not because of shame or frustration with Ellie, but out of a wish to shield her from this kind of torment. But this was only the tip of the torment.

For the most part, though, there was love and safety at Ellie's house. The same could not be said for school, where in today's terms she was a victim of bullying but in the terms of that time she was merely getting what she deserved. For instance, in seventh grade, the school nurse called a surprise weigh-in for all the middle-schoolers. Ellie was sent with all her peers from two entire grades to line up outside the nurse's office. Ellie knew this wouldn't turn out well; she dreaded it as she inched closer, becoming increasingly sweaty and nauseated. When she reached the doorway and the scale, the nurse eyed her with disgust. Ellie was then weighed. As she turned to leave, the nurse followed her into the hall, and though she hadn't done this with any other student, the nurse announced in full voice, "Weight, 268 pounds!" Needless to say, Ellie never forgot this moment of her life, and was never able to fully trust an authority figure again. "Safe places" were no longer safe. Not for Ellie.

That was only one of the many times Ellie walked the gauntlet.

Ellie continued to get larger each year, and as she did, she experienced increasingly horrifying responses. Kids would follow her down the street and heckle, and even sometimes physically accost her. It wasn't uncommon for mothers to point her out to their children, saying, "Look at the fat pig." Men driving by in trucks yelled obscenities. She was pummeled with beer and soda bottles, and for some bizarre reason, she was a dumping ground for ice cream and milk shakes. She was dehumanized, objectified, humiliated, degraded. She often felt she "didn't have a chance in hell as a member of the human race," and if she was seen as merely a fat pig, perhaps she didn't.

Her parents did try to intervene. First they attempted to speak to schoolmates' parents, which was a fruitless disaster. Then to teachers and school administrators. The attitude was unreceptive, perhaps because everyone seemed to believe Ellie brought this on herself. One year the school did bring in some type of counselor who was purported to be an expert in bullying. No, there was not a school assembly in which child actors portrayed the pain felt by the bullied, after which her peers stood behind her in solidarity. Instead about ten or fifteen fat girls, all girls, all fat, were brought to the guidance counselor's office and given a lecture on how they needed to take personal responsibility for the "attention" they were receiving. In fact, they were informed, they were obviously fat in order to elicit this attention. Positive or negative, attention is still attention, and these girls were asking for it. And that was that.

Quite a few girls accepted their self-imposed burden. Ellie didn't, but that was irrelevant to everyone except Ellie. For their part, the school was quite proud of its accomplishment, and the subject of bullying, in their eyes, was forever moot. As much as Ellie's parents wanted to help and made an attempt, they had little power over the world; they barely managed to control their own home. Conflict was the norm at the Fat Brunos', what with Ellie's father's hot mouth and the extended family imposition, not to mention a brood of fat children whom everyone else seemed to believe sealed their own fate.

If anyone was going to stick up for Ellie, it would have to be Ellie. She developed coping mechanisms. She learned to be witty and sarcastic; she was quick and cutting. And she learned how to spot and avoid the physically violent. That wasn't always an easy job, as violence would oftentimes arise from surprising places. For instance, unbeknownst to her parents (because she didn't tell), there was violence inside the family. Her uncle, her father's brother, began abusing Ellie when she was very small. It started out as emotional abuse and general cruelty, with a touch of physical abuse. When she was as young as two years old, her uncle would take Ellie's cheek in his fingers, and squeeze, and twist, holding on as hard and as long as he could. She would let out bloodcurdling screams. What others in the family thought was going on is impossible to image, but for reasons she will likely never know, no one came to her rescue. Later on, he began molesting her, and this continued for years, until he met his wife-to-be. She found out, although Ellie is not sure how or how much, and she made it stop. She was a savior to Ellie, and although the abuse itself is all very cloudy, that much is clear to her.

As brutal as the overt abuse was, the most devastating acts of all were much less dramatic. It is not the nature of the act alone that determines the intensity of impact. The identity of the actor is profound. As a very little girl, around two and three, she would wait for her father to come home after the night shift. Hers was the first bedroom closest to the front door. He would come in around dawn and she would greet him with a baby's love: "Hi, Daddy." A very sweet ritual, he would sit on her bed and give her a butterscotch or caramel from his pocket and spend a few moments with his first daughter. It was in many ways the highlight of her life. Her daddy was everything to her. Then one early morning her father, with no malice, just lack of forethought, gently poked her in her round three-year-old tummy and then pointed to her doll and stuffed bear. "He said, 'When you grow up, do you want babies like your dolly and teddy bear?' I said, 'Yes, Daddy.' He said, 'Do you want to get married and have children?' I said, 'Yes I do, I want to be a mommy.' He said, 'Well, no one is going to marry you and you're never going to have children unless you lose that weight, that stomach.' I was three years old. I didn't know what weight loss meant, I didn't know what fat meant. I just knew that by my father doing that, I was somehow defective." Ellie has never had children. She also has no more memories after that day of sitting with her father at dawn. She suspects they continued the ritual, but after that, all the memories faded away.

There were a couple of other times he did similar things. It was a regular practice for Ellie's father to go to his bedroom and read after dinner. She would follow him there and listen to what he read out loud. It didn't matter what it was, whatever he was reading. She just wanted to spend time with her father. Sometimes she would sit on his belly and bounce up and down and he would say, "You're making me sick." She wasn't, it was just daddy and his little girl being silly. One evening Ellie beat him to the bedroom and as he entered the room he looked down at her seven-year-old body and stated,

> "If you don't lose that weight by the time you're ten, you are going to have weight problems your whole life." That was another moment that shaped my self-esteem, and my relationship with men. I realized as I got older that he had his own issues and he was projecting. But if your daddy finds you defective...you know. Years later, I brought up those incidents with my father, and he denied them both.

Despite how large Ellie and her siblings were, it was not caused by what is so often blamed in present times. There was never junk food in their house. There wasn't money for it. Everything was fresh and homemade, and fruits and vegetables were always available. There was never a dinner without salad, even if all they had were celery and onions, there would be a salad with her father's vinaigrette. She didn't have a McDonald's hamburger until she was ten, and that was only because they were moving to a new house. Her mother, a religious coupon clipper, would on occasion bring home a box of cereal other than the store brand cornflakes, and even then it wasn't the kind with neon colors or mini-marshmallows. They drank gallons of ice water after coming in from playing, which they did every day until the streetlights came on. There was no money for ice cream. In fact there is really not much to say about the food they ate, except that by all accounts it was exactly what any doctor or judgmental busybody would recommend. There were the feasts, but certainly not every day. Perhaps there was a bit of urgency about getting a fair share, as the threat of there not being enough was ever-present. But it was not a house with abundance, and even if the children had wanted to be gluttons, it was a financial impossibility.

Ellie suspects that a great deal of her weight was genetic. It clearly ran in both sides of the family. There was also some element of protection that fat provided. Her uncle opened that door. But the torment of being fat was severe, so there was only so much that fat could do to ward off evil. Ellie also never had the kind of eating disorders that many people associate with being obese. She was never a binge eater, or bulimic. She was, though, starting sporadically in her teens, and later becoming life-threateningly severe, a "restrictive anorexic." This is exactly what it sounds like: Ellie starved herself—literally.

Eventually, Ellie did marry. She was in her thirties. She was nearly 400 pounds at the time, and she soon learned that her husband needed to have complete control over her, which included her body, and he encouraged her to eat in such a way that she gained a great deal of weight very quickly. Although Ellie wasn't a binge eater, she did enjoy the attention of being served food, and he would take her to glamorous restaurants and order her decadent meals. Ellie also enjoyed that there was never a sense of insecurity about whether there would be a next meal. There was always going to be a next meal. Her husband lavished her with food and other gifts. Not the gifts she wanted, or love, but food was a suitable substitute for her, for a while.

About halfway through their marriage Ellie was struck with pneumonia and was hospitalized. As she waited in the institutional hallway, unable to breathe, they acquired for her a bariatric bed. She was extremely large at that point. The bed had a built-in scale and she was instructed to sit on it and be weighed for proper treatment. She did not look at the scale, and made her way very carefully to the bathroom afterwards as they fitted the sheets. She was propped on the toilet, unable to stand on her own, and her husband came bounding in with a sense of excitement and glee. "Do you want to know what you weigh?" "No," she said. "Six hundred and seventy-nine pounds. *Six hundred and seventy-nine pounds!*" he said, seemingly thrilled. It was then she knew how much danger she was in—from her weight, yes, but mostly from her husband.

It was also then that Ellie started to become severely and chronically anorexic. She simply stopped eating. Eventually she lost over 400 pounds and nearly died numerous times. She came close to starving herself to death, and contracted several illnesses that resulted from starvation, including a a rare disease caused by malnutrition that left her with deep scars on her torso and legs.

It had actually been her plan to have weight-loss surgery, but she was already starving and the surgery was scrapped. Ellie spent a great deal more time in the hospital, and to avoid psychiatric commitment she began to see a therapist. Her therapist had never met an obese anorexic before, though Ellie knows quite a few. Severely malnourished and dying of starvation, Ellie was 300 pounds.

It isn't difficult to know why Ellie and her family were tormented the way they were. Fat people seem like obvious prey, and that is part of it. Tormentors tend to find easy pickings. The fact that there was a group of them as opposed to one individual was also significant, but not everything. They lived in an insular town, a bit *Peyton Place,* and the Fat Brunos weren't originally from there. The city motto was "Hometown Pride." Interpretations may vary. It was also a highly religious community, mostly Catholic. One wonders about the Christian tenets of tolerance and compassion, but it wouldn't be the first time—or the last. Whatever the case, all of the siblings were deeply affected. One of the brothers became a drug addict. At first, he used cocaine to lose weight. That spiraled, and he eventually overdosed, and died. There was a sister who died a few years before that. Ellie says she died of sadness.

As Ellie grew up, her mother never spoke of her own issues with her weight, and she never dieted or encouraged her children to diet. She died young, at fifty-six. She had stomach cancer and hadn't eaten for a year; by the time of her death she was 150 pounds. It was only at the very end, on her deathbed, that she admitted she had always wanted to be thin. The rampant torment that this entire family experienced solely based on their fat, and other people's perceptions of their fat, is nothing short of tragic. It's unfathomable that this kind of blind cruelty was inflicted solely because of the size of their bodies; and let's not confuse that with ill health from fat—which not a single person in the family experienced directly.

Ellie describes it as a cloud of oppression. "I will never say my, or my family's, problems were caused by fat. They were caused by hatred and fear and bigotry." How these things aid people in losing weight is questionable, at best. Those who think shame motivates have probably never been shamed, or have a sadistic wish for others to experience the pain they have experienced. Frankly, if shame successfully motivated fat people to get thin, there would be no fat people.

Ellie's father, always having a stubborn temper and a "hot mouth," has begun to open up about things that went on in the past. His brother, Ellie's abusive uncle, tried several times to kill him when they were children. Although the worst of the abuse Ellie experienced from her uncle had stopped earlier, Ellie only felt free at fifteen, when he, a vigorously devout Christian, greedily eyed her up and down in church and whispered, "You would be a knockout if you dropped weight." At 300 pounds and in skintight black jeans with snakeskin patches up the inner thighs, Ellie realized she felt nothing but contempt for him. And she already felt like a knockout.

That's not to say everything was smooth sailing from there. She experienced abuse in her life again, like from her controlling husband, who, ironically, wanted her to remain fat. Ellie eventually freed herself from that abuse as well. She did divorce him, though not before she deliberately gained 80 pounds in an attempt to save her marriage.

Most recently Ellie tried her hand at plus-size modeling. And with a great deal of therapy has gotten her anorexia and PTSD under control. She stopped taking narcotics cold turkey. She tolerates the physical pain resulting from malnutrition, so she can also feel the emotional pain, and mourn her sister's death. Now, at forty-five, she feels as though she is going through a rebirth. Ellie weighs just under 300 pounds, but that is of no consequence to her. Her health is all that matters. Yet she does notice that when she goes into a store no one even notices her. There are no leers or jeers; she is simply another person out in the world. So her physical health and her mental health are greatly improved. But it has been work, and she doesn't want anyone to mistake that the work has been about weight loss—because it hasn't. It has been about overcoming other people's perceptions of weight and the vicious ways they project those perceptions.

She says, "If everything I have been through hasn't stopped me, nothing can." There is no gauntlet she is afraid to walk through, now.

PART THREE

12

COLLATERAL DAMAGE IN THE "WAR ON OBESITY"

Programming Kids for Emotional and Eating Disorders

BY PEGGY ELAM, PHD

Dawn Friedman remembers her parents sitting her down when she was ten or eleven years old to tell her she was too fat.

"I don't remember the details," she wrote in the magazine *Brain, Child* in 2012. "I know it was summer, I know it was just before bed, I know we were in the family room—but I do remember my intense shame and the way my vision tunneled, as if I were looking through the wrong end of binoculars. I remember that I left the room differently than I entered it, as if my parts were strung together wrong and I didn't know how to operate my arms and legs."

Her parents' "loving intervention" led to Friedman becoming more self-conscious and less physically active, "afraid people were secretly judging me." In her teens she began alternately starving, bingeing, and exercising until she lost weight, but "could never believe what I saw in the mirror. My thinking around food became distorted. I lost my ability to know when I was hungry or when I was full or what I wanted to eat."

After meeting her husband in her twenties she slowly began eating regularly again, normalized her exercise routine, and gradually gained weight. By forty, she was fat and "still struggling (but closer) to finding peace in my own skin."

When her adopted daughter's well-baby checkup found the infant at the top of the height/weight charts at three months, the pediatrician accused Friedman of putting a bottle in her daughter's mouth instead of tending to her emotional needs, and wanted to put the baby on a diet. Fortunately, Friedman could easily see the birth mother's size and shape in her daughter's body.

"If she had been born to me," Friedman wrote, "I think I would have accepted the doctor's condemnation without question. I am used to thinking that my body is wrong." After carefully tracking her daughter's formula consumption, she determined the child was taking in about half the amount of formula per body weight recommended by the American Academy of Pediatrics.

Friedman changed pediatricians.

Eight years later her daughter was still at the top of the growth curve, "strong, confident, and healthy." And Friedman sees her and children like her facing "a new kind of danger. In a social climate where larger bodies are increasingly suspect, kids like my daughter are becoming public targets of disapproval, discrimination, and overt disgust."[2]

The War

In 1996 the US government, in a statement issued by former Surgeon General C. Everett Koop, declared a "war on obesity." As the campaign picked up steam in subsequent years, other surgeons general ratcheted up the pressure.

"Obesity is the terror within," Richard Carmona told an audience at the University of South Carolina several years ago.

---

2 Friedman, D. (Spring 2012). Weighing Down Our Children: The Battle Against Childhood Obesity. *Brain, Child: The Magazine for Thinking Mothers*.

"Unless we do something about it, the magnitude of the dilemma will dwarf 9/11 or any other terrorist attempt."[3]

The word *obesity* medicalizes fat bodies—that is, it implies all fat bodies are diseased even in the absence of health problems. *Obesity* and its companion word *obese* are rooted in the Latin *obdere*, which means "to eat all over, devour," and encapsulating stereotypes of all fat bodies becoming that way through gluttonous appetites.

When Carmona spoke at the University of South Carolina he had been calling "obesity" "the terror within" for almost a decade, sometimes in association with reports that "overweight and obesity" kill "300,000 people a year." Such blanket assumptions and the fear-mongering associated with them harm people of all sizes, but they especially hurt fat kids.

The Ammunition

In 1998 the International Obesity Task Force, a bariatric physicians' group that has relied heavily on pharmaceutical industry funding, was instrumental in advising the World Health Organization to lower the standards for categorizing bodies as "overweight." The IOTF was closely tied to the drug companies Roche and Abbott, which make the "anti-obesity" drugs Xenical and Reductil. The companies have been reported to have given "millions" to the IOTF.

Drug companies benefit from "raised public awareness" about "obesity" because it increases the market for their drugs, a representative of the IOTF told the *British Medical Journal* in 2006.[4] Widening the pool of people considered "diseased" also benefits

---

3 Associated Press (July 17, 2010). Obesity bigger threat than terrorism? Published online at www.cbsnews.com (http://www.cbsnews.com/2100-204_162-1361849.html). Others have reported Carmona calling "obesity a greater threat than weapons of mass destruction" as early as 2003.

4 Moynihan, R. (June 17, 2006). Obesity task force linked to WHO takes "millions" from drug firms. *British Medical Journal*, Vol 332.

others who sell "obesity" treatments by increasing the population of potential customers.

Funding the IOTF was a good investment for the drug companies. When the body mass index (BMI) categories were revised, millions of people who went to sleep in bodies considered "normal" woke up with bodies considered "overweight," without having gained an ounce. To maximize sales of products or services, it's not enough to simply widen the pool of potential customers for products or services. You have to convince customers they need to buy. Fear is a common motivator.

In 2002, William Klish of Texas Children's Hospital told the *Houston Chronicle* that if the "epidemic" of "childhood obesity" was not checked, "for the first time in a century, children will be looking forward to a shorter life expectancy than their parents." Three years later, the *New England Journal of Medicine* published a study whose authors attempted to support Klish's statement.[5]

Klish later acknowledged his statement was based on "intuition" rather than facts. The authors of the *NEJM* study also eventually acknowledged that their statement was based on "collective judgment" rather than scientific evidence.[67]

The retractions came too late and too quietly. The cry that the current generation of children will be the first to not outlive their parents has become a meme and one of the bullets in the "war on obesity."

In reality, life expectancy has increased dramatically during the same time period in which average weights have risen. From 1970 to 2005 average lifespan rose from 70.8 to 77.8 years, PhD

---

5 Olshansky, S.J., Passaro, D.J., Hershow, R.C., Layden J., Carnes, Brody, J., Hayflick, L., Butler,, Allison, D.B., Ludwig, D.S. (2005). A potential decline in life expectancy in the United States in the 21st century. *New England Journal of Medicine,* 352:1138-1145.

6 Gibbs, W.W. (June 2005). Obesity: an overblown epidemic? *Scientific American,* 292 (6).

7 Center for Consumer Freedom (March 17, 2005). Life expectancy: Another Obesity Myth Debunked. www.consumerfreedom.com.

nutritionists Linda Bacon and Lucy Aphramor report in a 2011 review of weight science in *Nutrition Journal,* and both the World Health Organization and the Social Security Administration project a continued increase in life expectancy.

That information seems to have escaped some physicians at the Centers for Disease Control.

Why does this matter? The concept that there is an "obesity epidemic"—one that kills hundreds of thousands of people a year and is especially endangering children—is used to justify waging "anti-obesity" and "obesity prevention" campaigns.

The Enemy

Fat is a condition of the body, not a behavior. It is impossible to separate people from their bodies. Thus the "war on obesity" is actually a war on fat people. This "war" is hurting many people, but perhaps none so much as fat kids.

The attempt to eradicate fat bodies from society is both born out of and increases moral panic. Moral panics occur when certain groups are considered a threat to society and demonized. "What about the children?" and "Save the children!" are frequent rallying cries.

"Childhood obesity prevention" tactics have ranged from improving school meals to removing certain foods and drinks from vending machines to weighing and measuring kids and sending "BMI report cards" (also known as "fat letters") to the parents of children deemed "overweight" or "obese." While some such actions are reasonable—who wouldn't want good meals served to schoolchildren?—others are patronizing, such as the assumption that parents must not have noticed their kids are fat.

The overarching problem with actions taken in the name of "childhood obesity prevention" and "treatment" is that they locate the problem in fat children's bodies, and thus identify the problem as fat children themselves rather than focusing on behaviors, environments, or situations that are problematic for all children.

Targeting fat children in health promotion campaigns not only fails children who aren't fat—as if it isn't important for all children, fat or lean, to be adequately nourished, move regularly, and live and play in safe places. It also blames fat children for actions taken in the name of "childhood obesity prevention" that will alienate and annoy most kids.

Why are birthday cakes and cupcakes no longer allowed in some schools? Fat kids. Why have the candy and soft drinks been taken out of some school vending machines? Fat kids.

In the United States, the moral panic about fat kids heightened as First Lady Michelle Obama chose "childhood obesity prevention" as her signature focus. Several eating disorders associations and other organizations and individuals have repeatedly urged Mrs. Obama to stop talking about "childhood obesity prevention" because of its stigmatizing effect, but her Let's Move! campaign still rides on the backs of fat children.

The Unintended Victims

From 1999 to 2006, hospitalization of children younger than twelve with eating disorders increased by 119 percent, the federal Agency for Healthcare Research and Quality has reported. Doctors have seen more young children engaging in unhealthy behaviors such as restrictive eating and purging after the children misinterpret messages aimed at fighting "childhood obesity" or observe their parents' weight-control actions, which are often cloaked in concerns about health.[8]

If they hear certain foods are "bad" or "unhealthy"—or, in our fat-phobic culture, "fattening"—children may stop eating those foods. If they hear that being fat is "bad" or "unhealthy," they think losing weight or maintaining thinness by any means

---

8   The Columbus Dispatch (July 18, 2011). More young children are alarmingly thin.

is preferable to being fat. These unhealthy practices can lead to malnourishment and eating disorders.

Fat kids may even earn praise for their unhealthy behaviors even though their weight loss may come with actual damage to their bodies.

Children are especially vulnerable to such issues during the transition of early adolescence, during which natural increases in body weight can collide with desire for peer acceptance and peer pressure to diet, triggering weight and shape preoccupation.

Three case studies published in the journal *Eating Disorders* by Canadian researchers in late 2013 illustrate how school-based "healthy weight" campaigns can trigger unhealthy behaviors in some children.[9] In each case, the youths' eating disorders were triggered by "healthy eating" or "healthy weight" programs in the absence of any preexisting concerns about weight, shape, or eating.

One fourteen-year-old boy became determined to be "the best" at "healthy living" when a "healthy living program" was introduced to his school. He began "eating healthy" and exercised an average of two to four hours per day, eating smaller and smaller portions and going to extremes to limit calories that were added to his food. For instance, he stuck his hand in boiling water to take out the tablespoon of butter his mother had added to a pot of pasta. After he became emaciated, his eating disorder was finally recognized and he was hospitalized.

A thirteen-year-old girl changed her eating and exercise habits after a dietitian's classroom presentation on "healthy eating." The dietitian had emphasized what foods students "should" be eating and what foods they "should" limit. The girl began restricting nutritionally dense foods, fats, and increased her physical activity. Six months after the dietitian's presentation, she was hospitalized with anorexia nervosa.

---

9 Pinhas, L., McVey, G., Walker, K.S., Norris, M., Katzman, D. & Collie, S. (2013). Trading health for a healthy weight: The uncharted side of healthy weights initiatives. *Eating Disorders: The Journal of Treatment and Prevention*, 21:2, 109-116.

Yet another girl developed anorexia nervosa after being assigned a school project on eating disorders as part of the health and nutrition section of her physical education program, and as a result started to worry about her own weight.

"Whereas healthy weight interventions are intended to promote health, they may not be risk free," the authors note. "These cases underscore the need to promote health, regardless of size, for all children and adults in the homes, schools, and neighborhoods they live in."

The Intended Victims but Unintended Consequences

Psychiatrist Jennifer Hagman, medical director of the eating disorders program at Children's Hospital Colorado, calls restrictive eating in formerly or currently fat kids "a new, high-risk population that is under-recognized.... They come in with the same fear of fat, drive for thinness, and excessive exercise drive as kids who would typically have met an anorexia nervosa diagnosis. But because they are at or even a little bit above their normal body weight, no one thinks about that."

"For some reason we are just not thinking that these kids are at risk," psychologist Leslie Sim, clinical director of the Mayo Clinic eating disorders program, told *USA Today.* "We say, 'Oh boy, you need to lose weight, and that's hard for you because you're obese'...when a child is obese and starts to lose weight, we think it's a really great thing and we applaud it and reinforce it and say it's so wonderful and now you're healthy."

Sim and some of her colleagues authored a September 2013 *Pediatrics* article reporting several cases of fat children whose eating disorders were missed by physicians treating them for associated problems.[10]

---

10 Sim, L. A., Lebow, J. & Billings, M. (2013). Eating disorders in adolescents with a history of obesity. *Pediatrics* 132(4), e1026-1030.

One fourteen-year-old boy had lost more than half his body weight while eating no more than 600 calories a day and running cross-country track in high school. But when he was evaluated by a pediatric gastroenterologist due to marked sinus bradycardia (a slowing down of the rhythm originating from the heart's sinus node) and dehydration, the possibility of his suffering from an eating disorder was dismissed.

Sim and colleagues report another child whose "obesity" was "identified and addressed" by her physician when she was twelve years old, prompting a succession of diets and finally a regimen of running seven miles a day while eating 1,500 calories a day. After a year of weight loss from the latter regimen the girl had stopped menstruating—a sign that her body fat had dropped below natural levels—and complained of dizziness and orthostatic intolerance, the development of symptoms when standing upright that are relieved upon sitting. Her physician prescribed birth-control pills for her amenorrhea and recommended that she drink more water. At a medical visit a year later—a year during which she had continued to lose weight—the girl's problems continued. Her mother expressed concern about her restrictive eating and minimal fat intake, but was ignored.

Six months later the girl again saw her physician for amenorrhea, though nothing was prescribed. Six months after that visit the teenager developed severe shin pain and was referred to a sports physician, who expressed concerns that she had developed the female athlete triad—eating disorders, osteoporosis (bone loss), and amenorrhea—and referred her for a sports nutrition consult. Amazingly, the dietitian recommended that she maintain her current weight and her disordered eating pattern.

Notes in the teenager's primary-care physician's records during this period indicated that "her BMI is currently appropriate" despite her mother's concern that she might have an eating disorder—a concern which turned out to be well founded.

As Sim and colleagues note, the physical complications of semi-starvation and weight loss are often misdiagnosed in fat or formerly fat children and teens, and attributed to rarer disorders. "Because of this misdiagnosis, referral for ED treatment is often delayed until the ED symptoms have progressed and physical and psychological sequelae are severe," they report. Primary-care physicians "need to be aware that youth with significant EDs can present at any weight," and that "any weight loss, even if it takes a child from overweight to the 'average' range, should prompt ED screening."

Eating disorders identification "should not hinge solely on weight status," Sims and colleagues emphasize. "Even in the absence of low weight, evidence of eating-disordered behaviors (e.g., driven exercise, rapid weight loss, extreme dietary restriction, binge-eating, compensatory behaviors such as purging), cognitions (e.g., unhealthy emphasis on the importance of weight/ shape, skewed or negative body image), psychological features (e.g., social withdrawal, irritability, rigidity) and physical sequelae of starvation should prompt immediate intervention and referral to appropriate services."

Prisoners of War

The physical and emotional symptoms of low weight include difficulty concentrating, worsening mood and irritability, extreme social withdrawal, cold intolerance, fatigue, bloating, and constipation. These symptoms were perhaps best demonstrated in the classic study on human starvation, the Minnesota Starvation Experiment, which was conducted on healthy male volunteers who were conscientious objectors to World War II.

As the men in the Minnesota Starvation Experiment lost 25 percent of their starting body weight, they exhibited changes in mood and behavior that eating disorders therapists and people with eating disorders would easily recognize, including increases in depression and severe emotional distress, trouble concentrating, declines in comprehension and judgment, hoarding behavior (of objects other than food), social withdrawal, and, understandably, preoccupation with food. One man who, along with all the other research participants, had been determined to be psychologically healthy before the onset of the experiment, cut off three fingers of his hand with an axe during the starvation phase, and was unsure whether he had done so accidentally or intentionally.[11]

It is informative to point out that during the starvation phase of this experiment, the men were fed about 1,560 calories a day. This amount is more than is recommended on many weight-loss diets.

While the men studied were not initially fat, losing a significant percentage of body weight can have similar effects on anyone regardless of their starting weight. As obesity researcher Jules Hirsch, MD, has pointed out, "If you take two women who both weigh 130 pounds but one used to weigh 200 pounds and one always weighed 130, they are not the same." The formerly fat person is likely to show the signs of starvation: lower metabolism, constant hunger, preoccupation with food, anxiety, and depression.[12]

It's not as if losing significant amounts of weight actually improves fat kids' health. "Overweight" teenagers diagnosed with "Eating Disorder Not Otherwise Specified" who lost 25 percent of their body weight but were not considered "underweight" enough to receive an anorexia nervosa diagnosis have been found to be more medically compromised than a comparison group of adolescents with anorexia nervosa.[13] Putting it another way: A group of fat teenagers who lost 25 percent of their body weight were in worse health than teenagers with anorexia.

It is normal for girls to gain weight and adipose tissue as they approach puberty. When they skip meals and restrict eating in

11 Keys, A., Brozek, J., Henschel, A., Mickelson, O., Taylor, H.L. (1950) The Biology of Human Starvation. University of Minnesota Press.

12 Leas, C. (). Fat: It's Not What You Think. (p. 73)

13 Peebles, R., Hardy, K.K., Wilson, J.L., Lock, J.D. (2010). Are diagnostic criteria for eating disorders markers of medical severity? Pediatrics , 125, e1193. Available online at http://pediatrics.aapublications.org/content/125/5/e1193.full.html.

efforts to lose weight or prevent weight gain, their efforts can permanently stunt growth and delay sexual development.

As far back as 1983—a decade before the "war on obesity" escalated—a study published in the *New England Journal of Medicine* described fourteen youths from nine to seventeen years old who failed to grow or to mature sexually because they were skipping meals and did not ingest enough calories in efforts to be slim.

Medical help had been sought for the youths because they were "late bloomers," not because the parents were worried about the youths' restricted food intake. Most of the children came from affluent families and homes where thinness was highly valued. "After the problem was identified, some parents were reluctant to offer more food," the Associated Press reported.[14]

The number one risk factor for developing an eating disorder is dieting, and yet weight loss is being constantly recommended to fat kids while weight control and fear of weight gain is promoted to lean kids. As eating disorders specialists and others have repeatedly pointed out over the past decades, "the more we're pushing the anti-obesity message, the more we're pushing kids into eating disorders."[15]

Six percent of youths suffer from eating disorders; 55 percent of high school girls and 30 percent of boys report engaging in disordered practices such as diet pills, vomiting, laxatives, fasting, and binge eating.

"In an adolescent culture of body loathing and weight obsession, disordered eating is often normative behavior," fat activist Lesley Kinzel writes. "This was certainly true when I was a kid and teenager, and given the ever-increasing obesity panic, I doubt things have gotten better since then. By the sixth grade, it was common for many of my friends to exercise for hours to make

---

14 Associated Press (September 1, 1983). Fat-fear may delay maturity. *The New York Times.*

15 Lynne Grefe, president of the National Eating Disorders Association, quoted in USA Today (September 2013?).

up for having eaten half a cookie, or to skip breakfast and lunch frequently in the hopes of losing weight, trusting that dinner with their families was enough to create the impression that everything was fine."

"Adolescents may be particularly vulnerable to the pairings of image and value that surround them in the media," psychiatrists Anne E. Becker and Paul Hamburg wrote in the *Harvard Review of Psychiatry* in 1996.[16] "They are avid consumers of imagery, desperately want to fit into cultural norms (albeit norms of a counterculture), and have not yet established a core identity strong enough to resist the impact of cultural image-making."

Young girls who are vulnerable because of early deprivation or trauma may be particularly susceptible "to feeling fragmented by adverse comparisons to prevailing ideals of body form and beauty," Becker and Hamburg note. For such a girl the pursuit of thinner bodies offers "some hope of control and success, in contrast to the problems in her family and the lack of easy solutions to them, the scars from psychological trauma, or the uncertainties in her peer relationships. For a vulnerable adolescent girl the visual media market a ready-made (if ultimately disillusioning) reformulation of her pain, an explanation for feeling bad about herself along with an action plan for taking charge."

That action plan? Lose weight, and become societally and medically acceptable.

Yet dieting not only can become a gateway to an eating disorder—it actually tends to make its practitioners fatter in the long run. Studies of children and adolescents have found that during three years of follow-up, dieters gained more weight than nondieters.[17]

---

16 Becker, A. E. & Hamburg, P. (1996). Culture, the Media, and Eating Disorders. *Harvard Review of Psychiatry.*

17 Field, A. E., Austin, S.B., Taylor, C.B., Malspeis, Susan, Rosner, Bernard, Rockett, Helaine R., Gillman, M.W., & Colditz, Graham, A. (October 2003). Relation between dieting and weight change among preadolescents and adolescents. *Pediatrics,* 112(4).

Eating disorders can be deadly. But conflating weight and health and assuming that fat bodies are inherently diseased can harm fat kids in other ways as well.

The *New York Times* reported in 2013 on the case of a plump, active six-year-old African American girl who died in 2010 after her pediatric endocrinologist attributed her "prediabetes" to her weight, encouraged diet and exercise, and applauded the weight loss that preceded the child's eventual organ failure and death. The girl actually had type 1 diabetes, in which the body does not produce insulin (the hormone that helps the body process the glucose it gets from food), not type 2 diabetes, in which the body produces insulin but becomes resistant to it. Type 2 diabetes can be managed through changes in eating and exercise. Type 1 diabetes can only be managed by providing the body with insulin.

The endocrinologist did not monitor her blood sugar, encourage the child's mother to do so, or alert the mother to danger signs of high blood sugar such as thirstiness and increased urination. When the child was finally so ill that her mother took her to a hospital, her blood sugar was five times the normal level, and doctors could not save her. In July 2013 a jury found the endocrinologist 100 percent liable for the child's death.[18]

Campaigns against "childhood obesity" frequently claim there is an "epidemic" of type 2 diabetes in children, which is actually rare compared to other problems. The incidence per 100,000 children of type 2 diabetes is 11.8—which means that no more than 11.8 cases of type 2 diabetes are reported per 100,000 children—whereas the incidence of autism is 340 per 100,000 and the incidence of eating disorders is 2,700.[19]

---

18 Samaha, A. (October 2, 2013). Type miscast: An Elmhurst doctor's type 2 diabetes misdiagnosis results in the death of a six-year-old girl. *New York Times.*

19 Merikangas, et al. (2010). "Lifetime prevalence of mental disorders in U.S. adolescents, results from the National Comorbidity Survey Replication -- Adolescent Supplement (NCS-A), *Journal of the American Academy of Child and Adolescent Psychiatry,* 29(10, 980-9; discussed

Eating disorders are 229 times more prevalent in children than is type 2 diabetes.

Rather than conceptualizing type 2 diabetes as an almost inevitable consequence of childhood obesity, type 2 diabetes is better framed as a response to genetics and oppression, nutrition professor and author Linda Bacon says. The endocrinologist who misdiagnosed the plump child with tragic results appears to have engaged in "BMI profiling," a term coined by psychologist Deb Burgard, an eating disorders specialist and one of the founders of the weight-neutral approach to health called Health at Every Size. (The Association for Size Diversity and Health trademarked "Health at Every Size" in attempts to prevent the term from being co-opted by the weight-loss industry. Or, as Burgard calls it, the weight-cycling industry, since most people who lose weight regain it—and often more—in two to five years.)

Hiding in the Trenches

BMI is calculated using a person's weight in kilograms divided by height in meters squared. Although the formula is widely used to categorize people as "overweight" or "obese," it does not actually measure or calculate the percentage of body fat and is not a good predictor of total body fat.

The formula was invented between 1830 and 1850 by the Belgian scientist Adolphe Quetelet, who used it to classify French and Scottish soldiers. Quetelet developed the BMI formula while trying to identify social deviants via what he considered to be physical abnormalities. The BMI formula was never intended as a means of classifying people for health purposes, or of classifying children.

The use of BMI as a health indicator has been criticized for all populations, but is especially problematic for children. Jon Robison, a health promotion expert with a doctorate in health

---

by Jon Robison, PhD in the *Absolute Advantage* issue *Helping without Harming: Kids, Eating, Weight & Health.*

education and exercise physiology and an MS in human nutrition, notes that children of ethnic origins that have shorter, denser body builds, such as Mexican and Navajo, are plotted higher on the BMI curve due to their naturally heavier weight even when they do not have more body fat than other children. Even more problematic, he adds, is that the most commonly used growth charts, published in 2000, are based on a previous, slimmer population of children and do not reflect that for more than a century children as a whole have been growing taller as well as heavier, and maturing earlier.[20]

When Katja Rowell was in medical school in the late 1990s, the total of her medical training in nutrition was a half hour on breast-feeding and a lunchtime lecture from a nutritionist. As a family physician, she advised parents worried about their children's weight with the standard, "eat less, exercise more" advice. When the children didn't lose weight, she assumed their parents were either lying or not following her recommendations. "I never asked myself if what I was telling them to do was actually helping," she wrote in her book, *Love Me, Feed Me*.

Then her daughter was born, a larger than average baby with a hearty appetite, and Rowell started researching nutrition, feeding, and children. One of the many things that surprised her was that as a group, the eating habits of lean and fat kids are pretty much the same.

"There's this bias we have," Rowell told Dawn Friedman for Friedman's *Brain, Child* article on the consequences of fighting fat in children. "I had it, too. I used to see a fat child walk by with a Starbucks drink with a bunch of whipped cream and think, 'Oh my gosh, what is that parent thinking?' What I didn't see was that his skinny brother was drinking the same thing."

Rowell supplemented her paucity of medical training on nutrition by delving into the research and studying under registered

---

20 Robison, J. (2007). Kids, eating, weight and health: helping without harming. *Absolute Advantage,* 7(1).

dietitian and therapist Ellyn Satter, a widely regarded expert on childhood nutrition, and became a feeding specialist.

Rowell told Friedman that concern about a "childhood obesity epidemic" is fed by misunderstandings about how children grow and what growth charts can and can't tell us. "Kids will do these periods of incredible growth and they're often preceded by weight gain," Rowell points out. "Sometimes kids will gain weight and kind of look a little bit softer and pudgier. Woe is the kid who shows up [for a checkup] right before their height spurt." Growth charts define children above or below a cutoff as unhealthy, when many children growing above or below average are doing well.

Rowell believes there is too much "obesity epidemic crisis" fueled concern about children's weight and eating. About a third of the clients she sees are parents of children under age four who are preoccupied (parents say "obsessed") with food, all of whom have been restricted for months to years in an effort to get them to eat or weigh less. She teaches and writes that children instinctively eat well overall when fed in a responsive, nurturing, and supportive way—and can grow up to be "eating competent." *Eating competence*, a term coined by Ellyn Satter and supported with research, is not about eating "perfectly" or "healthy" all the time, but rather being able to eat when hungry and stop when full most—but not all—of the time, and being able to enjoy eating without guilt or anxiety.

Competent Soldiers

When parents or professionals restrict children's access to food or brand certain foods off-limits in attempts to control children's weight or to promote "healthy" eating, forbidden fruit becomes more tempting. Children whose parents don't allow access to demonized foods don't learn how to enjoy them in moderation.

Rowell told Friedman about a six-year-old girl who snuck into a neighbor's house to find food she wasn't allowed to eat at home.

The neighbor found the child in the pantry drinking juice boxes and bingeing on boxes of crackers and cookies.

A Soldier's Alienation

Fat children are particularly susceptible to "anti-obesity" messages.

Kids think, "I am fat," not "I have fat," psychologist Deb Burgard told journalist Nancy Matsumoto during September 2013's Weight Stigma Awareness Week. Burgard has heard from many fat children who say, "When you talk about getting rid of childhood obesity, I think you want to get rid of me."[21]

Several years ago, a teenage girl told Linda Bacon that her school had recently started an "obesity prevention program" that included posters with the words "prevent obesity" on them. Every time the teenager walked by the posters she felt like she was getting kicked in the stomach—"like they're saying 'we don't want anyone to become like you,'" Bacon wrote in 2006. "She avoids a particular hallway because it always triggers bad feelings, and wonders what the campaign is doing to affect her classmates' view of her."[22]

The trauma of being identified as having an "unacceptable" body is not a new predicament, as adults who were once fat kids can tell us.

"I was always 'the fat kid,'" Charisse Goodman writes in *The Invisible Woman: Confronting Weight Prejudice in America.* "I wasn't me. I wasn't a name or a person, just an object described by an adjective. If I was naturally shy, I became doubly so.... I learned that no matter what anyone says, it really doesn't count if you're smart, kind, funny, sweet, generous, or caring, because if

---

21 Matsumoto, N. (September 2013). For Students, Perils of Weight Bias, Anti-Obesity Programs: Guidelines for childhood obesity prevention programs, exposing bias. Psychology Today website.

22 On the Whole blog (November 7, 2006). How campaigns to "prevent obesity" hurt those they purport to help.

you also happen to be heavy, you may find yourself on the receiving end of more cruelty than you even knew existed."[23]

In the comments on a *Dances with Fat* blog post about concern-troll bullying of fat children and adults, a woman posted that being subjected to bullying on the way to school gave her "an anticipatory stomachache every morning and prompted me to choose a path through the wood where a bear was known to den because that felt *safer*" than dealing with bullies. "How nice of them to give me a case of social terror that impaired my ability to hold down a job! All the therapy I poured money into to get over their crap was just a cost of living in the world the bullies own."[24]

Another woman commenting on the same post reported that as a result of being bullied about her weight as a fat teen she stopped cycling, roller-skating, and swimming for many years. "All that bullying did for me is make me unfit, unhealthy, and disinclined to deal with people face to face, all because I wasn't one of the lucky ones who could change."[25]

When therapist and college professor Cheri Erdman was a fat child, a kindergarten teacher encouraged her parents to send her to a residential weight treatment center for children with "special nutritional needs." She was five years old. During the more than a year she lived at the treatment center, her parents visited her once a week, on Friday nights.

Erdman's only clear memory of those thirteen months was of being on the playground and seeing her parents' car and her four-year-old brother Patrick beyond the chain-link fence.

"With longing we looked at each other from the prisons that separated us—a fence, a locked car, a camp for special kids, adults who thought they were doing what was best, and a society that

23 Goodman, W. Charisse (1995). *The Invisible Woman: Confronting Weight Prejudice in America*. Gurze Books.

24 Hansen, J. October 21, 2013). Comment on "Bullying For Our Own Good," Dances with Fat blog.

25 Pyctsi (October 21, 2013). Comment on "Bullying For Our Own Good," Dances with Fat blog.

was beginning to hate fat people so much that it had devised a place to put fat kids away until they lost weight," Erdman later wrote in her book *Nothing to Lose: A Sane Guide to Living in a Larger Body.*[26]

Psychotherapist Carmen Cool's earliest memory of hating her body occurred during Thanksgiving when she was in fifth grade. "I looked down at my stomach, gathered it up into my young hands, and said to no one in particular, 'I wish I could cut this off the way we cut the turkey.'"[27] The female family members around her laughed and agreed, expressing the wish that they, too, could cut off parts of their bodies.

Ragen Chastain, a dancer, educator, writer, and activist who blogs at DancesWithFat.com, was first criticized by her father for being fat when she was a preschooler. She stayed heavy even though she became a cheerleader, danced, and played sports. When she was seventeen, however, a family friend encouraged her to lose weight before starting college, and Chastain began dieting. She worked out eight to ten hours a day on 1,100 calories a day, finally collapsing while running on a treadmill.

She was hospitalized with an eating disorder. In the hospital, since she was eating adequately again, she started rapidly regaining weight. The weight gain concerned her doctors. As a result, while she was hospitalized for an eating disorder she was told she needed to lose weight.

It is a dirty little secret of the eating disorders field that some eating disorders specialists are biased against fat bodies. Such specialists, like Chastain's doctors, may encourage eating disordered behavior in fat people, not recognizing that such behaviors are as unhealthy for fat bodies as they are for thin ones.

---

26 Erdman, C.K. (1996). *Nothing to Lose: A Guide to Sane Living in a Larger Body.* HarperCollins.

27 Cool, C. (November/December 2007). Changing the Conversation: From "Preventing Obesity" to Promoting Health for ALL Children. *Absolute Advantage, 7*(1).

Stockholm Syndrome

Some "childhood obesity prevention" campaigns have attempted to shame children—and their parents—into losing weight and, ostensibly, improve health. In recent years Georgia's Strong4Life program employed images of unhappy fat children and a mother hanging her head in shame after her son asked why he was fat. "Stop Sugarcoating It, Georgia!" the campaign blared.

Sugarcoating what, exactly? Children as young as four already associate the word *fat* and fat bodies with negative stereotypes such as "dirty," "lazy," and "stupid." As psychologist Dina Zeckhausen told Atlanta's *Journal-Constitution*, "These words can form the basis for a lifelong shame-based sense of self. Such shame is at the core of addiction, depression, anxiety and a host of eating disorders."[28]

Stringent "anti-obesity" programs may sometimes lead to weight loss, but at the cost of increased eating disorders and emotional disturbances in the children targeted. For instance, Singapore significantly lowered the proportion of "obese" children in its population over the past couple of decades by forcing fat children to participate in daily strenuous exercise, feeding them less at lunch than their thinner peers, and insulting and shunning them. Such shaming and ostracism has "deeply scarred" the formerly fat children, a Singapore psychologist has reported, and the weight-focused program has been blamed for a sharp rise in rates of eating disorders and depression in the city-state.[29]

Fat children and adolescents hear the "othering" of the fat body by culture (and government, health care, peers, and family) and can begin to identify their own bodies as "others," demonized and dissociated. Dieting and other weight-loss pursuits become an attempted exorcism of demonized flesh.

---

28 Zeckhausen, D. (March 9, 2008). Childhood Obesity and the Schools: Shame hurts more than helps. *Atlanta Journal-Constitution*.

29 Zeckhausen, D. (March 9, 2008). Childhood Obesity and the Schools: Shame hurts more than helps. *Atlanta Journal-Constitution*.

But fat and flesh are part of the body, not actually alien to it, and bodies defend against perceived famine by slowing metabolism and driving post-famine eating and weight regain.

Despite fear-mongering about weight, health, and mortality, deaths from so-called obesity-related diseases such as heart disease and cancer have been decreasing over the past several decades, even as the weight of the population has increased.

The relationship between fat and diseases, including diabetes, is correlational rather than clearly causal. If many fat people have a certain condition, it does not mean that fat causes the condition. Instead, a third, underlying condition may cause both weight gain and associated health problems. Medications used to treat conditions may also cause weight gain. And, of course, many people gain weight *after* they become ill and less active, not before.

As researcher Paul Ernsberger, PhD, and others have pointed out, there are also many medical conditions in which fat people fare better than thinner people—a phenomenon known as the "obesity paradox."

The so-called war on obesity being waged on Americans and, increasingly, other Western populations, is an example of disease-mongering as well as fear-mongering. Disease-mongering is the practice of widening the boundaries of what is considered illness in order to expand markets for those who sell and deliver treatments for the "illness." Journalist Ray Moynihan and medical colleagues discussed the practice in a 2002 *British Medical Journal* article entitled, aptly, "Selling Sickness." "There's a lot of money to be made from telling healthy people they're sick," or "medicalising ordinary life," the *BMJ* authors note.

The term "morbid obesity," which is applied to BMIs higher than 40, is an example of disease-mongering and fear-mongering that has been absorbed into common medical parlance without awareness of its origins and original intent.

The term "morbid obesity" was invented in the 1950s by a bariatric surgeon named Howard Payne. Payne wanted to expand his weight-loss surgery practice, but back then such surgery was considered radical and risky. Payne figured that semantically associating death with a class of fat people would increase the likelihood of physicians recommending surgery for them. Now the term "morbidly obese" is commonly applied to very fat bodies, and bariatric surgeons are expanding the boundaries of the population they "treat" by encouraging such surgery at lower and lower BMI ranges.[30]

Disease-mongering and fear-mongering can harm by unnecessarily labeling people as ill or diseased, provoking poor treatment decisions, causing iatrogenic illnesses (illnesses that are caused by medical treatments), wasting money on unneeded products and services, feeding unhealthy obsessions with health, and distracting attention from sociological or political explanations for health problems. But such practices can be expected to continue as long as there is money to be made from whipping people into a frenzy about weight.

Redoubling Our Efforts

Current cultural attitudes and behaviors toward fat bodies operate on a framework of faulty assumptions about weight and health. Overarching this framework is a variant of what social psychologists call the Just-World Hypothesis—the belief or cognitive bias that people's actions always result in appropriate, predictable consequences.

Psychologist Melvin J. Lerner coined the Just-World Hypothesis after studying justice beliefs in the 1960s and observing the tendency of people to blame victims for their suffering. Lerner titled his 1980 monograph on the concept *The Belief in a Just World: A Fundamental Delusion.*

Belief in simple cause and effect and moral balance—that we can control outcomes through our choices and behavior, and that

---

30 Oliver, J. (2006). *Fat Politics: The Real Story Behind America's Obesity Epidemic.*

bad things happen as a result of people's actions and choices—is comforting in a capricious world. It can be terrifying to contemplate that bad things can happen to you at any time. As a result, some victims blame themselves to make events seem more controllable. For instance, the belief of many abused children and victims of domestic violence that they deserve to be abused may be a coping mechanism that allows them hope of warding off future abuse by changing their behavior.

This Just-World Hypothesis translates into beliefs that eating well (however defined) and exercising regularly will keep aging, infirmity, and death at bay and allow one to live the Good Life. Thus, people whose bodies meet societal ideals—ideals that currently in most Western cultures are slim, healthy, and youthful—are perceived as being better than those whose bodies do not meet the ideals.

No Justice in War

As psychologist Deb Burgard has pointed out, we can't tell how hard people work by looking at their bank balances. Neither can looking at the size of someone's body, whether child or adult, tell us anything reliable about his or her behavior.

Science confirms that weight or fatness is much more complex than the simple calories-in versus calories-out model that can be conceptualized as the weight-oriented version of the Just-World Hypothesis. The reality: Some people can become or remain fat while eating relatively little. Some people may be naturally inclined to be bigger than others.

Genetics is probably the most significant factor affecting weight. The heritability of weight is estimated to be as high as 70 percent. But there are many other factors scientists have found that affect weight and adiposity, including chronic dieting and weight-cycling, environmental changes, changes in food supply, pharmaceutical effects, endocrine disruptors, increased pollution, sleep deprivation, decreased smoking, and aging and maturation.

The "war on obesity" and "childhood obesity prevention" efforts are predicated on the assumption that there are safe, effective ways of permanently making fat people thin. But there is plenty of evidence that such efforts hurt more than they help.

The majority of individuals who participate in weight-loss programs regain virtually all of the weight that was lost during treatment, regardless of whether they maintain their diet or exercise program, Bacon and Aphramor report. Ninety-five percent of dieters regain the weight they lost, and often more, within three to five years. Even the few long-term studies of bariatric surgery outcomes show gradual post-surgery weight regain.[31]

Except at statistical extremes—extremely fat or extremely lean—BMI "only weakly predicts longevity," Bacon and Aphramor wrote in their 2011 analysis of weight science. "Most epidemiological studies find that people who are overweight or moderately obese live at least as long as normal-weight people, and often longer." Being fat is actually associated with better survival of many diseases.

There is little evidence weight loss will actually improve the health of fat adults and children in the long run. There's not even a way to test the hypothesis that losing weight will produce long-term health benefits, because there are not enough people who have maintained long-term weight loss.

In contrast, research shows that a high but stable weight is safer than repeated fluctuations in weight. Repeatedly losing and regaining weight damages the immune system and may itself increase the risk of heart disease and type 2 diabetes. Dieting has also been found to reduce bone mass and increase the risk of osteoporosis even in fat individuals, who generally are less likely to develop the condition. Dieting is also associated with increased psychological stress and cortisol production, both of which increase disease risk.

---

31 Bacon, L. & Aphramor, L. (2011). Weight science: Evaluating the evidence for a paradigm shift. *Nutrition Journal*, 10(9).

"Childhood obesity prevention" efforts operate under the assumption that fat kids eat more and move less than thin kids. But analysis of the reported dietary habits of more than 12,000 children and adolescents found that those who were clinically "overweight" and "obese" actually consume fewer calories than their thinner counterparts, beginning around age seven.[32] Researchers at the Johns Hopkins Bloomberg School of Public Health, examining activity patterns in US adolescents since 1991, found signs that in recent years physical activity among adolescents has actually *increased* while TV viewing has decreased. They found no clear evidence that US adolescents had become less active over the past decade.[33]

Unfortunately "childhood obesity prevention" campaigns may actually make fat children *less* active by making them more self-conscious about their bodies and increasing weight-related teasing. Weight-related teasing and body consciousness makes fat children, especially girls, more concerned about others seeing their bodies during physical activity and therefore less likely to engage in such behavior.[34]

Most fat children become slimmer as they approach adulthood. Children whose fatness persists into adulthood have been found to have no more disease risk as adults than do adults who have never been fat. The exceptions are fat kids who diet.

32 Hoyle, B. (May 11, 2010). Overweight & obese children eat less than their healthy weight peers. Medscape.com.

33 Johns Hopkins Bloomberg School of Public Health (November 2, 2009). Decrease in physical activity may not be a factor in increased obesity rates among adolescents. Press release.

34 Zabinski, M.F., Selens, B.E., Stein, R.E., Hayden-Wade, H.A. & Wilfley, D.E. (2003). Overweight children's barriers to and support for physical activity. Obesity Research, 11: 238-246.

War. What Is It Good For?

There is no "obesity epidemic," Linda Bacon and others have reported. The average weight of the American population has increased by just 7–10 pounds since 1991. During this period the average age of the population has also increased as baby boomers have grown older; it's natural for people to gain a little weight as they age. And even that small increase in average human weights has leveled off.

Interestingly, although this slight increase in average weights has been attributed to increased food and sweetened-beverage intake and more sedentary lifestyles, along with other factors discussed above, a similar slight increase in average weight has been reported in laboratory animals—whose eating and exercise patterns have not changed over the years—as well as in some wild animals, none of whom, we can assume, are more likely to indulge in junk food and Big Gulps than their ancestors.

The "war on obesity" is being waged in the name of health, but in fact is anything but healthy. There's also little evidence that the war is accomplishing what it intends: reducing the incidence of "childhood obesity."

One eight-year-long study costing $20 million followed 1,704 third graders in forty-one elementary schools. Some of the schools were randomly selected to be left alone, while others received the intervention: reduced-fat breakfast and lunch meals, "healthful" snacks, classroom lessons on "healthy eating," educational programs for parents, and having the children participate in physical exercise for an hour at least three times a week.

"At the end of the study, the students could successfully parrot back their nutrition lessons, and the cooks could successfully prepare low-fat meals, but, as reported in the *American Journal of Clinical Nutrition*, 'The intervention resulted in no significant reduction in percentage body fat,'" Connie Leas reported in *Fat: It's Not What You Think*. A similar study following more than 5,000 children from ninety-six schools in California, Louisiana, Michigan, and Texas produced similar results.

War Blindness

The National Institutes of Health, which sponsored the two large studies, has acted as though the studies never existed. Instead, the NIH has started a new program called "We Can" that is intended to change children's diet and increase their exercise.

As Leas reports, that's not all bad. "Exercise is a good thing. Removing soft drinks from the schools is a good thing. Vegetables and fruits are good things. But the focus of 'We Can' is clearly on getting children to lose weight, equating being thin with being healthy. And, predictably, their nutritional information lists fat as a 'WHOA' food (food to be avoided). Even though the huge studies on school children showed that reducing their fat intake did not result in thinner kids, the 'We Can' program still casts fat in its old demonic role."

For her *Brain, Child* article Dawn Friedman interviewed David Katz, MD, founding director of the Yale University Prevention Research Center and senior medical advisor at Mindstream Academy, a Bluffton, South Carolina, co-ed boarding school for "obese" teens. Katz told Friedman that the fat children he sees at the boarding school are in an "existential crisis."

"They are asking, can I fit into this world the way it is? Can I live? Can I function? Can I be happy? Every day they wrestle with those questions and most days the answer is no."

Fat kids are miserable, the argument goes; they would be happier if they were not fat. Therefore, they should be helped to lose weight in order to be more acceptable to the world around them.

"In an enlightened age where we are having (mostly) reasonable discussions about transgender kids, anti-racism, and bullying in general, this attitude stands out," Friedman writes. "Rather than promoting tolerance, the accepted approach with obesity is to tell fat kids that they're the ones who need to change."

As I write this in late October 2013, a North Dakota radio station has reported that a female caller claims she's not handing out Halloween candy to children she considers "moderately obese." Instead, she's giving fat kids a letter to give their parents in which she tells parents it's "irresponsible" to let their fat children trick or treat.

An eating disorders expert told the local ABC news affiliate that singling out fat children in this way is a really bad idea. Local residents agreed.[35] Most of the online comments to an article reporting the woman's plan recognized it for what it was: bullying.

In a survey of a thousand British youths ages seven to eighteen conducted for the television program *Dying to Be Thin: Tonight*, which aired in January 2012, 28 percent of children less than ten years old and 44 percent of the eleven to thirteen age group had been bullied over their weight. Related, more than one in four children in the seven to ten age group reported they had skipped a meal in hopes of losing weight, while 45 percent of the eleven- to thirteen-year-olds reported having dieted.[36] More than a quarter of the kids surveyed reported having visited anorexia websites. One in seven reported being on a constant diet. Sixteen percent thought laxatives are a good way to lose weight.

Sometimes bullying and weight-related teasing come from family members. When the parents of fat children make negative comments about their weight, the children are left without any place in which they are accepted unconditionally.

One woman interviewed by attorney Sondra Solovay for her book *Tipping the Scales of Justice* reported that her father, "a world-renowned doctor, quipped that he wished I would 'catch anorexia' and then took it to the next level when I was older by stating flat out, 'I'm ashamed to be seen with you.'"

Parents who have internalized self-hatred after years of chronic dieting may pass that self-hatred (and fat-hatred) on to their children. "Fat parents can be extremely oppressive about fat and food issues," Solovay notes. "They may be desperate to make

---

35 ABC13. (October 30, 2013). ND woman handing out letters, not Halloween candy to kids she considers 'overweight.'

36 HuffPost Lifestyle United Kingdom (January 8, 2012). Bullied children under 10 turn to diets to cope with weight anxieties.

their children slim to help their kids avoid the harassment and lost opportunities they learned about firsthand."

Teasing about weight by family members appears to have even more of a negative impact on teen girls than does weight-related teasing by peers, researchers at the University of Minnesota have found. Their study of 2,516 adolescents primarily from inner-city schools found that more than a third of "overweight" girls engaged in extreme weight-control behaviors such as vomiting or taking diet pills or laxatives to lose weight. A history of being teased about being fat was one of the strongest predictors of risk for being "overweight" five years later, as well as for engaging in "extreme dieting." Family-based teasing had twice the effect of that from peers.

"Most families where there is weight-based teasing are not abusive," lead author Dianne Neumark-Sztainer, professor of public health at the University of Minnesota, reported in a media report of the study. "They just don't realize how hurtful it is. These findings show that your home needs to be a safe haven."[37]

The Rubble

In her dissertation research examining comments on fat acceptance blogs and interviewing fat individuals, Lonie McMichael, PhD, found that many fat adults report that when they were children, their parents told them they must lose weight to be acceptable. Some of McMichael's research participants reported being forced to play sports to lose weight and being complimented when starving themselves.[38] Some parents and other relatives have encouraged fat kids' dieting, or tried to camouflage fat kids' bodies to make them appear thinner, in efforts to avoid social judgment for having fat kids. Women are often blamed when their kids are

---

37 Newswise (September 20, 2007). Many overweight teens have same eating disorders as thin peers.

38 McMichael, L. (2013). Acceptable Prejudice? Fat, Rhetoric & Social Justice. Pearlsong Press.

fat, reports Glenn Gaesser, PhD, author of *Big Fat Lies* and direc-tor of the Exercise and Wellness Program and Healthy Lifestyles Research Center at Arizona State University.

Parental focus on children's weight also interferes with chil-dren's development of internal regulation of eating—what feeding specialist Katja Rowell refers to as eating competence. Ironically, attempts to restrict children's eating have been found to acceler-ate weight gain in those children.

Even if fat children's homes provide safe havens from negativ-ity, they still risk exposure to the toxins of fat hatred whenever they step outside.

"It is hard to feel adequate, let alone proud of yourself, when everywhere you look, there is literally a sign saying there's some-thing wrong with you," journalist Kate Harding wrote on her blog *Shapely Prose*.

A member of Lonie McMichael's research focus group said that when she was in the second grade, a boy punched her in the stomach and knocked her down. When asked why, he said, "I hate her because she's fat." So, she said, "I learned early that the world was dangerous for fat people."

Even the Boy Scouts of America are not safe places for fat kids. The organization banned Scouts with BMIs of 40 or higher from attending their Jamboree in 2013, expressing concern that the boys' assumed health problems could not be addressed adequate-ly where the Jamboree would be held. Boys with BMIs between 32 and 39.9 were required to provide extra health information to the Jamboree medical staff.

In criticizing the organization's actions, the National Association to Advance Fat Acceptance reported a 2009 incident in which a boy was dieting and trying to lose weight in order to attend a Scout adventure camp. The boy's mother told NAAFA that her son played football, wrestled, lifted weights, swam, and participated in several track-and-field sports, but he was deemed too heavy (and ostensibly too unhealthy) to participate in the camp. The boy had been conditioning himself for the camp for two months by hiking for two to three hours wearing a 50-pound pack and eating only 1,200 to 1,400 calories a day in an attempt to lose weight.

"I am concerned that the emphasis on childhood obesity is having a backlash," Susan Ringwood, chief executive of the Eating Disorders Association in the UK, told a *Times* reporter in 2007. "We know people who are bullied about their shape are far more likely to develop eating disorders, and there is now even more focus on overweight young people."[39]

Body weight is one of the most common reasons for bullying—more common than bullying due to race, religion, or disability, with rates similar to that of bullying due to sexual orientation, researchers at Yale University's Rudd Center for Food Policy and Obesity reported in the journal *Pediatrics* in January 2013.

On Cordelia Moon's first day in gym class at a new high school, the gym teacher measured her fat with calipers, over Cordelia's objections. The teacher then told Moon, "loud enough for everyone to hear, that I had the highest body fat of the class!" Sondra Solovay reported in *Tipping the Scales of Justice.* "The teacher went on to say it was surprising because I didn't 'look that fat,' but suggested I start a restricted-calorie diet immediately.'"

After the class, a girl told Moon she was relieved to no longer be "the fattest in the class."

Moon never returned to the gym class.

As noted earlier, school "healthy eating" programs may inadvertently trigger eating-disordered behavior in students. School staff may also model unhealthy weight-control practices. In meetings of the Boulder Youth Body Alliance, one teenager reported that "our nutrition teacher said today that when she wants to lose weight, she picks up smoking for two weeks."[40]

---

39 Yeoman, F. & Bennett, R. (February 3, 2007). Antiobesity message 'is driving girls to anorexia.' *The Times.*

40 Cool, Carmen. (2007).

Weight-based victimization increases the risk of binge eating, unhealthy weight-control behaviors, increased preference for sedentary activities, and skipping physical education classes—all of which, the Rudd Center researchers note, can lead to weight gain. Of course, bullying is problematic even if it doesn't contribute to weight gain; it can lead to low self-esteem, depressive symptoms, suicidal thoughts and behaviors, skipping school, and poorer academic performance.

Researchers have found that aerobic fitness is more important than weight in predicting academic performance on math and reading tests in fourth- to eighth-grade students.[41] All the more reason for schools not to support weight-based "health" and "childhood obesity prevention" programs that make fat kids more self-conscious and inadvertently discourage them from participating in physical activity.

The Rudd Center researchers who studied weight-based victimization were particularly concerned about the high percentage of adolescents who reported that their parents teased them about their weight. "Research indicates that weight-based teasing from multiple sources (e.g., peers and parents) may be associated with increased emotional health problems for youth," they wrote. "Even well-intentioned parents may inadvertently criticize or tease their overweight children in ways that are extremely damaging."

Tragedy Is Inevitable

A ten-year-old Illinois girl described as "overweight" committed suicide in November 2011 because she was being bullied about her weight.[42]

---

41 Rauner, R.R., Walters, R.W., Avery, M. & Wanser, T.J. (August 2013). "Evidence that aerobic fitness is more salient than weight status in predicting standardized math and reading outcomes in fourth- through eighth-grade students. J Pediatr, 163(2). 344-8.

42 Matthews, L. (November 14, 2011). Ashlynn Conner, 10, allegedly commits suicide because of bullying. International Business Times.

A fourteen-year-old UK girl hanged herself in July 2011 after complaining that girls at her private boarding school were taunting her about being fat. Her parents say she had become bulimic as a result of the taunting.[43]

A twelve-year-old Florida girl committed suicide in September 2013 after being bullied online by several other girls for nearly a year. After she climbed a tower at an abandoned concrete plant and jumped to her death, police searched her computer and found queries for topics including "what is overweight for a twelve-year-old girl."[44]

A fifteen-year-old Connecticut boy killed himself after the first day of the 2013–2014 school year due to being bullied for being tall, heavy, having acne, and being from Poland. "Despite the abuse, the family thought he had turned a corner in the past year," a news report stated. "Having lost weight and even making some friends, they thought he was finally starting to fit in."[45]

Fat children are more likely to be bullied than are children who are not fat, independent of gender, race, family socioeconomic status, social skills, and other factors. Children who are teased about their weight are more than 50 percent less likely to do well in school compared to peers who are not teased about their weight.

Can We Rebuild?

When researching her *Brain, Child* article on cultural attitudes toward childhood "obesity," Dawn Friedman asked nutrition

---

43 BBC News Somerset (June 2012). Fiona Geraghty inquest: Coroner attacks fashion industry and media.

44 FoxNews.com (October 15, 2013). Girls, 12 and 14, arrested in death of bullied Florida girl who killed herself.

45 Gorman, R.(August 30, 2013). 'If I stabbed myself, would anyone miss me?': Tragic message of boy, 15, who killed himself on the first day back at school 'because he couldn't bear being bullied by classmates again.' Mail Online (http://www.dailymail.co.uk/news/article-2407001/Bart-Palosz-Connecticut-teen-kills-day-school-bullied.html).

professor and author Linda Bacon if she believes the mainstream perspective on fatness will ever change. No, Bacon said—there's no money in accepting fat bodies.

"Who would need mascara if you believed your eyes were beautiful without it?" Bacon asked. "Everyone has a stake in our self-hatred."

Rational strategies to managing threats to one's perception of a Just World include accepting that injustice exists, trying to prevent injustice or assist victims of injustice, and accepting one's limitations. Where fat kids are concerned, such rational strategies include acknowledgment that weight-based health promotions and "childhood obesity prevention" campaigns increase dangerous dieting behavior and inflict other harm in children and teens.

Weight-focused health campaigns, including "obesity prevention" programs, encourage restrictive eating behavior that alienates kids from their natural appetites and from their bodies as a whole. It doesn't matter whether the recommended practice is called "lifestyle change" or "healthy eating"—if the goal is to alter weight, it's a diet. Dieting has been shown to contribute to compulsive eating and eating disorders as well as emotional disturbance. Chronic or repeated dieting also actually causes weight gain by slowing down metabolism, and sets kids up physiologically and psychologically to crave and binge on the foods they have been denied.

> "We shouldn't focus on weight, per se, but rather on other factors that may be the underlying causes of disease like physical activity, social inequality, and stress," sociologist Abigail Saguy, PhD, told the Robert Wood Johnson Foundation's *Human Capital Blog* in late 2013.

One way to enhance the ability of all kids, including fat ones, to thrive is to make sure all health interventions and public health campaigns focus on lifestyle and safe, healthy environments rather than weight.

"Weight is not a behavior and, therefore, not an appropriate target for behavior modification," Sigrun Danielsdottir; Deb Burgard, PhD; and Wendy Oliver-Pyatt, MD, authors of the Academy for Eating Disorders' *Guidelines for Childhood Obesity Prevention Programs*, point out. Therefore, they say, interventions should be referred to as "health promotion" rather than "obesity prevention," since "the ultimate goal is the health and well-being of all children, and health encompasses many factors besides weight."

Other recommendations in the AED guidelines include that terms such as "overweight" and "obesity" and anti-fat messages such as "fat is bad" should be avoided due to their propensity to promote weight-based stigma. Children should be weighed only when there is "clear and compelling need for the information," and then only in a private setting and "recorded without remark." Unhealthy weight-control efforts should be screened for while protective behaviors such as mindful eating, positive body image, and decreasing weight-related teasing and harassment are promoted. Efforts should be focused on making children's environments healthier rather than only emphasizing individual responsibility. (For the full AED guidelines, see the Academy for Eating Disorders website at www.aedweb.org.)

Psychiatrist Leora Pinhas and colleagues at the Hospital for Sick Children in Toronto recommend sensitivity training for adult role models like teachers to help them avoid transmitting their own biases about food, weight, and shape onto children and youth. In addition, they stress, messaging around health should be common to all body types and be accompanied by school rules preventing weight-based teasing and other weight bias.

"Helping children learn to appreciate their bodies for what they can do, rather than how they look, may help to reduce feelings of self-consciousness or embarrassment that may prevent participation in activity," Marion F. Zabinski, PhD, and colleagues recommend in reporting research on barriers to physical activity for "overweight" children. "In addition, helping children reduce the value of shape, weight, and overall appearance in self-worth will be central for improving body image."[46]

The data are clear. In order to ensure the well-being of fat kids and the adults they will become, we must reframe the focus of "anti-obesity" campaigns from "preventing" or changing certain weights to focusing on good nutrition, physical activity, and healthy environments for *all* children.[47,48] It's time to cease fire in the "war on obesity" and address the damage it has done.

Peggy Elam, PhD, is a clinical psychologist and publisher. After earning a bachelor's degree in journalism, she worked as a newspaper reporter, editor, and columnist for several years before earning her master's and doctoral degrees in psychology from Vanderbilt University. Her psychotherapy practice included a focus on eating disorders and trauma survivors. In 2003, she combined her literary and psychology expertise to found Pearlsong Press, which specializes in fat-positive fiction and nonfiction and promotes health and happiness at every size. More information on Dr. Elam can be found at PeggyElam.com.

46 Zabinski, M.F., Selens, B.E., Stein, R.E., Hayden-Wade, H.A. & Wilfley, D.E. (2003). Overweight children's barriers to and support for physical activity. Obesity Research, 11: 238-246.

47 Hayes, D. (February 7, 2012). Strong bodies, smart brains: promoting healthy weights for all kids in schools [unpublished lecture notes]. Nutrition File Seminar 2012, Edmonton Marriott at River Cree Resort, lecture cited in Chute, J. (June 2012). Emerging topics in weight management: Challenging conventional wisdom. *Nutrition File for Health Educators.*

48 Robison, J. (Ed.) (November/December 2007). Helping Without Harming: Kids, Eating, Weight and Health. *Absolute Advantage: The Workplace Wellness Magazine, 7* (1).

13

MEASURING THE CAKE

Hannah's mother was an avid baker, and a good one at that. There would always be cakes and cookies and all types of delectable Southern sweets in the fridge and the cupboards, tempting, if not calling out to be devoured. Frostings and glazes. Creamy and crisp. The lushness of butter covering the tongue. Or the snap of a wafer slightly gritty to the teeth. Sugar and vanilla, cinnamon and nutmeg, lemon, orange, hazelnut. Chocolate! Wafting through crevices, floating under doors. Who can resist such glorious temptations? But that was the test. The test of willpower, and more importantly, obedience. Even a sliver gone was noticed, in fact it was calculated, measured, and each part subtracted from the sum of the whole. And with every morsel unaccounted for, shame and regret.

It was sadistic. It was control. It was devastating. It was merely an extreme version of what many people go through with food every day.

Hannah was raised basically in the middle of nowhere. She lived with her mother and father, and a brother who was three years younger than she. Her mother was stricken with some kind of mental illness, though never defined. She was filled with anxiety, narcissism, and terrific mood swings. And though it wasn't easy to label, she also had eating disorders and a distorted perception of her body. Her body defined her. Whether that was a direct consequence of mental illness is not clear, but what is clear is that mental illness, body image, and food were twisted into some warped vicious battle, and Hannah was an extension of that in her mother's eyes. It eventually became an extension in Hannah's own eyes, as well. There really was no escape.

Hannah was not a fat kid. Perhaps a bit plump. To her mother, though, she reflected fat, and fat was just about the worst thing one could be. The irony was that her mother, a born Southerner who cooked like the Southern best, would do so as a regular course. It would have been difficult not to develop a sweet tooth in that house, as everything that filled the shelves was designed to do just that. And to be a trap. It was the regular practice of Hannah's mother to count every item, weigh, and measure. Each day she would set about measuring the cake. It was a ritual. She knew the precise amount that had been there the day before, and the precise amount that had been removed. And if there had been any removed, Hannah experienced her wrath.

Hannah was put on Weight Watchers, for the first time, at age seven. It was a must she be put on the program because her mother was adamant that "no one will ever love you if you are fat." Perhaps even worse than lack of love in her mother's view, her mother was certain there are no fat cheerleaders. Hannah never wanted to be a cheerleader, but that was beside the point. It was perhaps symbolic. The more distorted it all became, the more Hannah did actually gain weight. The verbal abuse became proportionally worse. While in the midst of cooking and baking the temptations—the callings—Hannah's mother would tell her daughter that she looked as if she could live forever on her fat.

So Hannah became a closet eater. She literally would take food into the closet to hide and eat it. It was how she handled the stress. The verbal abuse was simply more than she could take. She developed a "great dislike" for her mother, and thus started a sort of cat and mouse game, with both Hannah and her mother being cast as the cat. Hannah would try to outsmart her mother, the satisfaction of the win outweighing the repercussions of the loss. She would examine the Tupperware, then take the tiniest sliver of cake from one side and the tiniest sliver from the other, making sure they were precisely the same. Then she would replace the lid and the container exactly as they had been. Hannah would eat the cake and wash the dish by hand, placing it and the utensils just where she had found them. She barely got a taste of the cake; the enjoyment was more in the trickery, which she often pulled off. This was the greatest of capers and height of rebellion. Outwitting her mother's control was a satisfaction in childhood that had no rival, and was a major topic of discussion in therapy for years to come. To this day Hannah will take matching slivers from cakes, though there is no one to hide it from.

Hannah's mother enjoyed being a martyr. She would cook these elaborate foods and barely take a taste, and when she did, she would berate herself, often proclaiming, "I am a hog." Then she would lament her figure, which was perfectly normal by any standards, except her own. She never seemed to binge or purge. She wasn't anorexic. She had what might be an eating disorder "not otherwise specified." Food was Hannah's mother's worst enemy and she craved it desperately. She would sit and read cookbooks and magazines with pictures of food. Lounging in a chair, she would pore over the ingredients with what could only be described as lust. It seemed normal to Hannah when she was a child. Today, though, Hannah despises cooking. She loathes using a recipe.

Then there would be diets. When Hannah was in high school, her mother would prepare diet food for them both. Steamed fish and vegetables. Though her mother wasn't overweight, she perceived herself as such and hated her body. She projected that hate onto Hannah. At the same time as the dieting, her mother would continue to bake, continue to count, continue to measure, and then, the foods would mysteriously disappear. Her mother would blame the disappearance on Hannah and her brother. It was an added demented twist, seeding the doubt between them all. Who was guilty? Who deserved to be blamed? Who deserved to be punished?

Then Hannah lost 50 pounds. She didn't try to, she was just busy with friends and spending time out of her closet. She became the golden child. She was lavished with praise. Not for her good grades or for being a good person or for having a good heart, only for having less fat. Hannah didn't buy it, but that didn't stop the twisted game or efforts to control. Hannah's mother had a misguided belief that Hannah lost the weight to please her. She didn't. When the cookie count or the cake circumference would remain the same Hannah would be praised. She knew this wasn't normal because her friends' mothers didn't measure the sweets. There was no daily analysis or intervention for them.

But next, Hannah went to college, where she gained weight. Though she didn't go home much, when she did, she would be reminded about how much weight she had gained—as if she didn't already know—and Hannah developed an eating disorder. Hannah became bulimic. She would binge out of control, after which she would feel horrible and induce vomiting as well as take laxatives. That went on for a few years until she was hospitalized for low potassium. At the time, it was conventional wisdom that anyone with an eating disorder had been sexually molested—that becoming fat was protection from abuse, and care could only be properly given in a psychiatric hospital, so that is where Hannah was sent. Hannah was also medicated for good measure. She began the process of trying every diet available, losing then gaining more, and repeating the process. The hospital and their medication offered no cure, though when she got out, she was slightly slimmer.

Then Hannah got married. She was only twenty-two at the time she met him and she weighed about 180 pounds. She felt she looked good. But despite making a commitment to him, which included wedding dress fittings with her mother, she realized she wasn't in love with the man. That didn't stop the wedding plans, and in the course of the preparations, Hannah gained 100 pounds. She is uncertain if it was a result of stress or a test of his love for her, but it certainly made visits to the dress fitter with her mother horrifying. By the time she became pregnant with the first of her two children, Hannah weighed 333 pounds. They have now been married for twenty years and it has been more than a decade since he has touched her. If her body size was a test of his love, he has failed. However, they are the best of friends and he is committed to the marriage otherwise, as is Hannah. Except for the affairs.

And then Hannah's mother got breast cancer. Mother was young, in her late fifties, and despite Hannah's childhood, there was a part of her who wanted to please her mother, and she lost 87 pounds. Her mother died feeling as though Hannah was the golden child. On her death bed, she told everyone about the weight loss, an affirmation of her work as a mother. After her death, Hannah gained it all back, and more.

Hannah's final effort to lose weight came with lap-band surgery, not too long ago. It all started at age seven when Hannah's mother, dissatisfied with her own body, decided Hannah was fat and needed to diet. Over the course of the next decades, and dozens of diets, Hannah gained and lost and gained again enough to actually become fat, many times over. And now, finally, the surgical intervention. Her mother had passed by this time, but by now that was irrelevant. So she went to a clinic that specialized in weight-loss surgery, took a mortgage on her house, and had a lap band inserted. Hannah lost 10 pounds and became, for the first time, sick from being fat. Technically, sick from the lap band, but to those who judge her, what is technically true is merely trivial.

She is heavier now than before the surgery and cannot eat many foods. No vegetables and fruits, or the kinds of foods that maintain a healthy body. She has lost chunks of hair and has debilitating migraines. She is unable to work and has gone on disability. The headaches are so bad, she is a regular at the emergency room, fearing an aneurysm. Once she was transported by ambulance to the ER directly from her doctor's office—he was at a loss for what to do. Though her lap band is no longer functional, she cannot find anyone to remove it. They fear another surgery will do greater damage. Her surgeon has lost his license and the clinic refuses to help her. A lawyer has advised her to sue.

Hannah is trying to put her life back together. She wants to be healthy; she also knows by now that being on a restrictive-calorie diet results in her being heavier, in the long run. It's been proven to her, over and over. Hannah has adopted a paradigm called HAES, or Health at Every Size. The fundamental premise is to focus on health rather than weight. It does not proclaim that every fat person, or any person for that matter, can be healthy— just that health is the goal to strive for rather than a number on a scale. With HAES, any ailments are treated independently of weight and there is no diet, in the weight-loss sense, but people aim to eat a healthful diet and use their bodies to the best of their abilities through various types of movement and exercise, preferably in a form that someone enjoys. It is becoming increasingly popular as people realize that traditional diets do not work for them and it may be possible to be healthy in a larger body.

Hannah has come to realize that the only people in her life who have been truly judgmental of her size have been her mother, and herself. She has been successful in school and career and prides herself as a pretty good mom to her children. Though her marriage is not ideal, her husband does not judge her weight. She has come to realize that what is physically attractive is subjective. There is not much one can do about it, other than find someone who likes you the way you are. She and her husband do care for each other, though not romantically, and remain best friends.

That's not to say Hannah likes being fat. She hates paying for two plane tickets and it's uncomfortable sitting in a car or a small chair. Doctors still lecture her, though what they expect her to do, since she had done everything, is unclear. She reads a great deal about size acceptance and works to undo the damage that began at such an early age.

Hannah has two children—her son is seventeen and her daughter is fourteen. Neither of them is overweight in the least, but that didn't prevent food issues. Her daughter was treated for anorexia. At five foot six inches and 99 pounds, she passed out at school and admitted to the nurse that she hadn't been eating. She had been hiding her skeleton with baggy clothing, but that's not to say it went unnoticed. Hannah noticed, but her husband was in denial, and because of Hannah's past, she was terrified to say the wrong thing about weight. Hannah has never pressured her children one way or another; in fact, she never mentioned weight to her children at all as they grew up. Of course they knew she was overweight, but the kids never mentioned it. It's possible Hannah's daughter harbored some fear that she might end up like her mother, but Hannah suspects is was mostly social pressure that led to the anorexia. Her daughter wanted to be skinny in her skinny jeans; at a size 0, she felt like she had earned something laudable.

Hannah arranged treatment, and her daughter is improving. The greatest motivator for the girl was her wanting to run track. Her BMI was so low that she didn't pass the physical. And she had no energy. Even at fourteen, she understood this was not good. It has never become clear what prompted the eating disorder exactly. Perhaps her daughter doesn't know. Perhaps we all underestimate the power of peer pressure and social cues. Perhaps the unconscious connection between a mom and her girl is so strong that this sort of thing happens by osmosis. Perhaps when her daughter gets older, she will understand, and let Hannah know.

Hannah did diet around her kids, though she certainly never suggested they do so. Still, just watching the behavior of counting out twelve chips has to send a message. They claim that Weight Watchers is based on healthy lifestyle change, but is it healthy to ration crackers and save up for a piece of birthday cake? Is our obsession with food and thinness so ingrained that we no longer know what is normal? Perhaps that is why her daughter became anorexic. Perhaps it's everything together in the pressure cooker we call a teenage brain.

Hannah's daughter went to outpatient treatment so she could continue regular school. Interestingly, though disturbingly, her friends knew about the treatment and it didn't faze them a bit. The school counselor allowed kids in such treatment to eat in his office, if they had concerns about eating in public. He also allowed them to bring a buddy, and it became sort of an exciting game: Who would get to be the eating partner in the private room? Eating issues were not new to these children, and that had nothing to do with Hannah. It's simply ubiquitous.

So Hannah, during her lifetime, witnesses two extremes: The fat child forced to diet by her parents, and the thin child who was never encouraged to watch her weight at home, but was still subject to societal pressures. The outcomes, it seems, are not that different. It turns out the extremes are not that extreme. The result of clear emotional abuse, and merely living in a culture obsessed, are both devastating. Whatever the source, a focus on weight, diets, size, thinness, fear of fat, and the need to control, leads to dysfunction.

When they were children, Hannah's brother was a bit chubby too. He also got berated, but never to the same extent as Hannah. Hannah was a girl, of course, and it was different for girls. Hannah's mother, in her own twisted sense of reality, believed her intentions, and thus her actions, were pure. She wanted Hannah to wear pretty clothes and date pretty boys. Hannah's mother was doing all this for Hannah's own good. She was training her for life, and the most important lesson to be learned was that of avoiding temptation, by any means necessary.

Of course, the best way to instill a lesson is in a real-world situation, and family gatherings offered the perfect opportunity. On Thanksgiving, which seems to be a great day for teaching, the family would travel twelve hours to visit. Everyone would bring some kind of food, and Hannah's mother would prepare her specialty: luscious sweets. One particular year a dessert had been made in advance, and not knowing it was explicitly for the holiday, Hannah and her brother ate some pre-trip. This demanded a lesson! The pan was brought to the festivities with the chunks missing and presented to the family, with the added explanation that it looked as it did because, "My children ate it like dogs."

Hannah and her brother were humiliated, and rightly so, at least according to the lesson plan. The family didn't know how to respond, so they did nothing. In adulthood, when Hannah's mother had long died, her now-grown cousins brought up these lessons. Of course it was a little late.

Though it may have been hard to tell, Hannah did have a father in the picture. In fact, he was right there in the house. Although Hannah adores him (he lives with her now), he did not protect her. He never stopped the persecution, the accusations, the humiliation. Although she loves him, she resents him as well. At times she has felt his silence was tacit agreement, that he was disgusted by her too. He never said so explicitly, but then again, he didn't say much. They have never discussed it, never addressed Hannah's anger for his inaction, his lack of protection, his own fear of Hannah's mother and the recrimination he would have faced if he had been heroic, or even less than stoic. They have also never discussed, and still never discuss despite him living in her house, his alcoholism. Decades of drinking. Self-medicating. Willful ignorance in a bottle that allowed him to be blind, deaf, and dumb to the abuse. He is still a drinker. He is still not ready to talk.

Outside of her relationship with her father, Hannah does talk, though sometimes she is afraid. She started talking about weight with her brother and all the damage her mother's obsession had done. She talks to her children. She is concerned that her daughter worries she will turn out like Hannah. But perhaps like her own father, Hannah fears she might say the wrong thing. When Hannah mentioned to her daughter that her dress size is a 28, it was beyond the child's comprehension. The girl didn't know clothing was made in that size, and larger. But Hannah feels it is essential her daughter understand that people are different, and under no circumstances should her girl learn from Hannah to hate herself, as Hannah's mother taught. Hannah doesn't push. Even at the worst of the anorexia, Hannah was never angry, never forced her daughter to eat. She only offered support and concern for her health. Just her health. That she should grow up to be physically sound, be able to have children, have no residual illness. It was a double-edged sword, that support. Health is always the way in when people show concern about weight. "I just care about your health." It can seem like a trick.

Primarily, Hannah aimed to express to her daughter that size does not characterize a person. Whether it's a size 0 or a size 28, a body size does not define an identity, or direct happiness. At least it shouldn't. That is such a narrow way to view a life and so much is missed. Hannah has good days, and still sometimes, bad. But she has worked not to let her body make or break her, and she attempts to teach her daughter the same.

It was a strange reality among her daughter and her peers when she was anorexic. Although Hannah is unaware of her daughter's friends suffering from anorexia, clearly they had insight from somewhere. They all took it in stride. Just another day. Just another eating disorder. While Hannah's daughter had developed extreme anxiety eating in front of most people, she felt no discomfort when her girlfriends enthusiastically joined for a glamorous private dining experience in the counselor's office. It seemed almost a badge of honor to be chosen, and at the very least, a welcome break from the daily routine. No one seemed to be concerned a stigma might attach to them. No fear that they might appear to be the one ill, somehow defective or an outcast. It appeared that from the perspective of teenage girls, going through the eating-disorder treatment process was the norm, and, daresay, even cool.

Hannah had also received treatment for an eating disorder when she was a teen, though not anorexia. It was more of a vague fat disorder that people seemed to think she had, though she weighed only 155 pounds. It was different then. At nineteen, she was pulled out of college and sent to a facility. She had inpatient treatment for six weeks. And then the insurance ran out, and miraculously, she was cured. It was an unfortunate miracle, because in point of fact, Hannah loved being there. She could speak freely and wasn't judged. She could talk about her mother, she could tell the truth.

There were no eating disorder units back then in her small town. Hannah was placed in a psych hospital with women having all sorts of conditions—some eating disorders, also suicide attempts, depression and anxiety, and those with borderline personality disorder (as identified at the time). It was the regular course of treatment to bring the family in for therapy, but Hannah didn't want her mother having any part of it. Hannah suspected the therapist, at first, didn't quite believe her mother stories. Hannah was "going off the rails." So the therapist brought Hannah's mother in anyway. In complete character, Hannah's mother was angry and embarrassed for being blamed, and took no responsibility for the dynamic. This prompted Hannah, for the first time in her life, to tell her mother to "fuck off." Her mother jumped out of her seat in a fury and threatened to smack Hannah in the face, right in the middle of family therapy. There were then the apologies typical of an abuser, and myriad calls and letters. Hannah disregarded them and the therapist summed it up: "Your mom has some issues."

There was never a "come to Jesus" moment between Hannah and her mom, and after Hannah returned home, the eating disorder, the threat, and the psych hospital were never mentioned again. Her mother, it seems, conveniently forgot it had ever happened, most likely in the hopes the nosey neighbors would also forget. She had an image to maintain.

But Hannah didn't forget. She actively does not forget. It isn't lost on Hannah that issues with food and weight continued as a pattern with her own daughter, and although Hannah never overtly displayed any of the destructive behaviors her mother did, she wonders what she might have subtly and subconsciously conveyed. At the same time, she recognizes that food and weight issues are a societal condition, beyond our individual control.

There is this whole attack on childhood obesity and I think it is going to backfire, the same way it backfired for all of us who were put on diets and sent to fat camp. It's going to cause eating disorders, it's going to cause worse outcomes, bullying and self-hatred. I see it as a disaster in the making. It's never been easy to be a fat kid, or a fat adult, but what goes on in our culture today, the media, I really believe with all my heart and my experience that instead of focusing on the obesity epidemic that kids should be taught to love themselves unconditionally, that they are good people the way they are, that what you have to offer society does not depend on the size of clothing that you wear. I feel like I have to do twice the work not to be judged, not to be seen as lazy and unmotivated, and it is a struggle to overcome the same thoughts I have about myself.

The struggle with weight isn't easy, it's not just about pushing yourself from the table. There are emotions involved, heredity, and factors beyond our control. To see that passed on to my own daughter, the same ideas, even though she wasn't even fat to begin with, just shows me the epidemic isn't about obesity, it's about obsession with weight. It's everywhere. I grew up with a sadistic mother and my daughter is growing up with a sadistic culture. The end result seems to be the same.

14

CONVEX

Each Thanksgiving Day there was a ceremonial cutting of the pies. The matriarchal grandmother of the family would ring in the event by assessing who would be bestowed the three-inch slice, and who in turn would receive the half-inch sliver. By age five Sandy was henceforth assigned her place in the family. She belonged with the sliver eaters, because she, and they, were fat.

Actually, as is so often the case, when you look back at pictures of Sandy as a child, she wasn't so much fat as she was merely fatter. She was fatter than her two younger sisters, whose bellies were so flat you could see the outline of their ribs. Not that they were too thin, necessarily, they were just built to be more concave. On the other hand, Sandy had a round belly. She was convex. Though, the matriarch would not have gone in for geometry metaphors. Thin is thin and fat is fat, and as far as she was concerned, that is that.

As it was, Sandy was about kindergarten age when her grandmother honed in on her round belly. From that day forward Sandy was a fat one, and the family rules for fat people applied to her. About half of Sandy's extended family was fat, and they all were expected to live by the rules assigned to fat people, or so her grandmother would have it.

Sandy was a surprise. Much to the matriarch's chagrin, Sandy's young parents were dating. When Sandy's mother came up pregnant the grandmother was certain that her saintly son could not be the father. He was being trapped by a shameless strumpet; the child was not his. Nonetheless the two were married, and Sandy was the spitting image of her daddy. His sisters had prayed for this, as in fact, Sandy's mother was a good catch. She was kind, and she was slim. It was Sandy's daddy who was the fat one of the pair, and Sandy was his spitting image. Still, it never seemed the matriarch fully took to Sandy, her disdain shifting from the seed of Sandy's birth to the roundness of her stomach.

This wasn't lost on Sandy, and she, too, was unhappy with the size and shape of her body. It made no sense to her; her sisters were so thin. It also made no sense that many of the adults around her seemed to think this was entirely within her control. When she would exercise, her chest would hurt terribly and she couldn't breathe. They would tell her she was out of shape and lazy and to run more, work harder. She was thirty before she was diagnosed with asthma.

It's not that her parents weren't loving; they were, very much so. But her mother was always worried. Why would just one of her daughters be fat? She was thin herself. But fat is relative. Sandy was five foot nine inches tall by high school, with long, skinny legs and plump in the middle. She looked like a giraffe. It wasn't bad, but it was different.

It was mostly the matriarch who was aggressive about Sandy's need to change her shape. She bribed Sandy with money, thirty dollars (a good payday at the time) if she could get into a size 10 by the end of the sixth grade. Sandy tried the cabbage diet. It lasted two weeks. Her mother, a dieter herself, was passively complicit, but it was kept a secret from her dad. He had strong beliefs about food as well. Three meals a day and a clean plate. When he finally noticed that Sandy would merely move her food around and not actually eat it, that was the end of that. Not that she could have kept it up anyway. No one can live on cabbage alone.

Also, food, eating, size, and health were a complex issue for all in the family. Just several years earlier, Sandy's mother had been showing signs of illness. At around the time of the cabbage diet, she was diagnosed with multiple sclerosis. As Sandy's mother became more ill, not fat to begin with, she lost weight. It was the only benefit of her disease, she said. A message confusing for anyone, especially a twelve-year-old girl with a round belly.

Dad, it has seemed, had a very different attitude toward life. He was a pastor, an amateur opera singer, and a sight to behold. He loved to dress and always donned a crisp suit or sporty jacket and slacks. His six-foot two-inch, 350-pound body—spit-shine-proud—was a beacon in their little town, and those surrounding. When not stirring a crowd with one performance or another, he would travel on a trusty motorcycle to visit his flock, bringing wisdom and comfort in a massive but dapper package coming through a puff of smoke. Though his mother the matriarch doted on him otherwise, she was not pleased about his size. No matter, he was a pillar of steel and Sandy's mother, despite her own body issues and those she projected onto her daughter, thought he was the most handsome man in the world. Embarrassing Sandy and her sisters terribly, Mom would swoon over Dad. Watching him ride on his motorcycle she would sigh to the girls, "My goodness, isn't your father sexy."

Sandy's mother had no issues with her father's size—in fact she seemed to admire it. He was strong and that meant safety. Also a woodworker, he would build things in his spare time. He hiked. He once broke up a 50-pound oak office chair for firewood with his bare hands, when most anyone would use an axe. He was a mountain in motion. So it was surprising that he was always desperate to lose weight. Or maybe it wasn't. The doctors would tell him if he didn't lose weight he would die from fatness. The media had begun its obsession with fat; Phil Donahue seemed to be constantly yelling in the nation's ear: "You have to be thin!" And then there was the matriarch; she always had an opinion.

Her dad didn't press Sandy, but again, in this family, different people had different rules. Just a few years after Mom was diagnosed, Dad was one of the first in the area to have a stomach stapling, and he was never the same. He got terribly sick afterward, and though he never discussed it, he lived with uncomfortable and embarrassing stomach problems for the rest of his life. To add insult to injury, though he lost weight for a time, it was not long before he gained it all back as well. He was only fifty-nine when he died. He had a mild cancer but died from an immune system weakened by the drugs they used to cure it. It is not clear if the illness associated with the stomach stapling contributed to his weakened immune system. It is clear that his weight was not directly his demise.

For many years after her father's death, Sandy thought she would never have weight-loss surgery. Not because it made her father sick, or perhaps hastened his death, but because he had gotten fat again. Because it didn't work. That is how powerful her drive to be thin was, the only thing she seriously considered is whether it worked.

There was really no other clear voice in Sandy's life when it came to weight. Her father, though he never criticized her, demonstrated his feelings about fat with his actions. And through her own dieting, so did her mother. But of course the strongest voice was the matriarch. She was the thin one of three sisters, the thin one, and therefore, the pretty one; the thin one, and therefore, the self-disciplined one. She believed that weight was entirely within a person's control, and sharing that insight by whatever means necessary was generosity. Granted, at the time, and even now, most people feel giving tips to the fat is generous. She also believed, as most people still do, that no one who is fat could possibly be happy. It's true that being a fat kid made Sandy unhappy, but it wasn't her body size that was the primary culprit. She was told in no uncertain terms that as a fat person, unhappiness was to be expected, and deserved. No other possible reality occurred to her.

The annual Thanksgiving pie ceremony was not as straightforward as it appeared. A subversive plot was afoot, filled with subterfuge. Sandy remembers it well and with great affection. She was not the only fat person in the group of thirty or forty guests that the matriarch held court over. In fact, about half of them were fat—she was just the youngest. With her initiation into the subculture came a new ritual. On Thanksgiving morning, each year, her uncle would steal a pie. After dinner when everyone was going about their business watching football and napping, young Sandy and her uncle would sneak to the attic stairs and celebrate the holiday together, with their secret stash of pie. It made Sandy feel recognized, special, loved. One could view it as a sad and desperate gesture, one that might even lead Sandy down a dark path of secret food consumption. But that is not how she remembers it. For her, it was all about inclusion. Camaraderie. Acceptance. It wasn't until Sandy was an adult that she realized her uncle was no more than ten years older than she when he perpetrated that caper. That made the memory even more special: He lived through and could understand the alienation—they were two children together fighting the system, even if just for a moment in time. That's not to say it wasn't heartbreaking they were relegated to eating their pie in the attic. Because it was.

It's not that the matriarch offered her love only conditionally, but the thin were treated differently from the fat. The thin relatives were permitted to simply live. The fat ones had additional expectations, and motivational incentives. "If you lose weight I will give you this, or let you do that." Fat was a barrier to normal life, by design. Fat was also a reflection of character, and striving to improve that character was expected, which meant actively working to be less fat. When on a diet, there was a certain leeway permitted. Dieters are "trying." Trying, regardless of outcome, was tolerable, but not trying was a crushing disappointment. So perhaps the love was conditional. But the matriarch believed these expectations to be just. Noble even. Her good intentions overrode the pain she caused, she thought. And there was pain. But the matriarch did not invent this worldview; it was pervasive. And still is.

Sandy's parents, while not promoters of the matriarch's ways, did not intervene: She was who she was, immovable, ubiquitous. When in the room, her personality dominated. Though when she left, there was an excited air, even frenetic. The teacher had left the classroom and spitballs would fly. Nevertheless, that didn't undo the damage.

Sandy could never quite wrap her mind around her mother's attitude toward Sandy's weight. Her mom was perpetually concerned with her own figure, though she was always slim. And she seemed to worry about the impact being fat would have on Sandy later in life. Although she didn't exactly press it, she was always encouraging when Sandy attempted to diet. There may too have been a subtle nodding of the head when the matriarch would harp on Sandy's weight. Her mother, it is fair to surmise, was conflicted on the matter. At the same time that she would support a weight-loss plan, Sandy's mother would also let her know she was beautiful and talented and could be anything she wanted to be. Perhaps she was simply a product of our culture. Sandy's mother loved and supported her daughter, but fat was scary, it seemed the entire world insisted it would ruin a life—and since she loved her, Sandy's mother certainly didn't want ruination for her daughter.

However, much scarier, Sandy's mother, it turned out, had a very fast-moving form of multiple sclerosis. Within two years, she was walking with a cane, and by the time Sandy was finishing high school, mom was using a motorized scooter. She became so busy battling her disease that parenting got whittled down to the essentials. Interestingly, in terms of attitude and perspective, she became a far better parent. No longer did Sandy's mom see Sandy as flawed for being larger. No longer did she project that body size was an issue. To her mother, Sandy, and all the girls, were the most perfect specimens on earth, in every regard, and no one could tell her otherwise. Sandy's mother clearly had gained new insight, and this was also around the time Sandy found surprising enlightenment of her own.

Prior to her seventeenth year, Sandy spent each summer with the matriarch, and each of those summers she was put on a diet. At seventeen, though, Sandy was sent to her other grandmother (her mother's mother), who had recently undergone surgery. She hadn't had the pleasure of much time with this grandmother previously. But the two grandmothers looked alike, both were slender and full of energy. This is what Sandy expected of grandmothers, as well as a contentious attitude. Much to Sandy's surprise, not all grandmothers were alike, and this one shed an entirely new light on the world, particularly when it came to nurturing, unconditional love, and delicious food.

For one, this grandmother didn't believe dinner had been properly served unless there was dessert. Every day, Sandy and her grandmother would happily prepare the evening meal together. They would plan and execute it, and both thoroughly enjoyed the process. Plus, this grandmother was a fantastic cook. There was always some homemade goody to close out the meal, and it would be designed to suit the supper. Sandy had never thought of such considerations. It might be a cake for hearty fare, or Jell-O for a light meal. It was orchestrated, joyful, and completely new to Sandy. There was certainly no planned dessert at the matriarch's house. "The fat ones didn't need it and the thin ones could get their own." Most interesting to Sandy was that her mother had been raised by this woman, by such a strong personality, yet she had long ago learned to appease the matriarch. Whether intentionally or not, Sandy's own home reflected the matriarch rules, plus with her mom being sick, the daily focus was on coping, not meal planning.

Also new to Sandy, this grandmother was a fitness buff. She was manager of the local YMCA and actually swam every day. During that summer, Sandy became a member and was permitted to take all the classes she wanted. Sandy went swimming three times a week and took aerobics, by choice. It was not like dreaded gym-class aerobics in school, where Sandy would get bullied for even trying. This was fun. There were all sorts of people, all sizes and ages, and while they would sweat together they would laugh. For the first time in her life, Sandy understood it was possible to like exercise, and she did.

Each day, Sandy would trek to her great-granddad's ranch. He was ninety-five at the time and still living in his same tiny house. With her grandmother laid up, it was Sandy's job to fix him lunch. There was only one rule: It had to have gravy. She could fix him anything, but there must be gravy. As he had done every day of his ninety-five years, he used the leftovers for the morning's cold gravy on toast. Tradition. Satiated, he would go out and tend to his garden, after which he would dart around the ranch on his four-wheeler, and inexorably get lost. He loved his life, and this was the first time Sandy witnessed that the road to longevity didn't demand perfection. He would talk and talk about this and that, while he smoked his ever-present pipe. There was no judgment with these people, just the ups and downs of living, and having as joyful a time as possible while doing it.

It was that summer Sandy decided which type of person she wanted to be. It was that summer Sandy learned there was a choice.

In actuality, this revelation was not altogether a positive experience. Sandy became quite angry, and for a long time. The bitterness she felt toward the matriarch and that entire side of the family—for not only singling her out as a problem and treating her differently, but also for perpetuating negative feelings she had toward herself—was difficult to process. It all seemed unjust, and unreasonable.

But out of this anger, Sandy came to realize that ultimately, she could be responsible for her own life choices, and she chose to be a person she liked, though she also realized she did not have complete control over her health and certainly not her genetics. For many years, she continued to diet, believing still that thinness was the route to health and happiness. Sandy was a vegetarian for twenty years, and even a vegan for some. She was still bombarded with messages from the outside world that fat was inherently unhealthy. Though ideas on how one ceases to be fat continued to change. For a long time, it was believed that any fat in foods made one fat in body, hence her decision to give up meat. And then there was a cosmic shift and carbs were the devil. All bets were off. It has been a solid twenty years of craving Kentucky Fried Chicken, which required an enormous amount of willpower. Realizing that, she never again considered a fat person to be lacking willpower.

By this time, Sandy had children of her own, and how to raise them, given her genes and her history, was a quandary. The last diet she attempted guided her to the answer. A faithful dieter, she followed the program and exercised more and more each day. Yet inexplicably, she was still gaining weight. Sandy had been able to lose weight on diets in the past, but not this time. She understands it now, but at the time it was truly shocking. She, as most people are, was still under the false belief that losing weight was a simple mathematical formula: Calories in versus calories out. She knew nothing about a body resetting its homeostasis so that it would retain the fat, as a body does with great aptitude. But if for whatever reason diet and exercise didn't work, enough was enough. Sandy quit dieting.

It was about then that Sandy began to read about the Size Acceptance movement and alternative perspectives on weight and health. It was good timing, as her two youngest children were just around the age of puberty. Her daughter, who had always been thin, started to fill out and become round—in all the right places, and some considered not so right. Initially, it was difficult for Sandy, the messages about thin were deeply ingrained. Her own experience as a young woman informed her that too many curves, especially say, around the belly, were not nature, but rather, problems. Exploring size acceptance ideology offered Sandy a new way to interpret women's bodies and helped to provide a focus for her daughter other than the skewed ideals Sandy knew growing up. This didn't assuage all of Sandy's concerns; there was still fretting about her child's wardrobe and external influences that were certainly not enlightened or empathetic. But Sandy was determined that no negative messages would come from home. At least she had control over that.

Then, as if the thin-obsessed universe was fighting back, her son began to put on weight. This was a few years prior to puberty and he was significantly larger than his sister had become. Sandy says he looked like the token fat boy in every pal movie, the Tubby or Fatso, presumably ribbed in a loving way, only to have a heart-wrenching scene where he expresses the pain of being an outsider. He had been quite thin until that point, even thinner than his sister. When he started to gain, family members felt it proper to point it out: "Isn't he getting kind of fat?" Previously slim, her kid was now round with a double chin, and Sandy, once again, was faced with the dilemma. Is there a problem here to address?

According to his school, there was a problem indeed. At the height of Michelle Obama's Let's Move! campaign, his school was weighing and calculating BMIs of all the students. Within the first two months of his high school freshman year, not only was a letter sent home informing the parents their child was obese, but the information was also posted on the Internet. The school, in all its thoughtfulness and concern, had a "Parent Center" webpage. Under the "Health" tab was included all the children's weight, BMI, and other fatness-related information. They somehow neglected to include vaccinations, allergies, special physical needs, or any actual health-related material. But it was apparently important that every parent be aware who was fat, electronically in writing. Needless to say, Sandy was angry. But systems are difficult to fight, and as she had with her daughter, she made sure home was a safe place. Sandy educated her son about weight, health, and whether there are correlations between the two. That was something he certainly wouldn't learn in school.

Like Sandy, her son also has asthma, but unlike her, his was recognized early—his difficulty breathing was noticed on their hikes. Given an inhaler by his doctor and a note for PE class that he was permitted to use it, his breathing issue was not blamed on being fat and lazy, and he, unlike Sandy, loved gym class and playing sports. The boy's most proud day as an adolescent came when he broke his hand wrestling with friends. With nothing to be ashamed of, he gave it his all, and was awarded the cast of honor.

Sandy's husband was actually the first to come to a revelation about the children's size. He, too, had become fatter as he got older and hated his Santa-like form. He tended to be self-effacing and Sandy would discourage derogatory words about his own belly, especially in front of the kids. In short order, he trained himself to be kinder. As such, it was easier for him to accept his son for who the boy was becoming. So everyone in the family, through their changes, simply went on as normal. They continued their family activities, hiking trips, and all things outdoors—fat or otherwise.

Sandy additionally worked hard on decriminalizing food, so to speak, which did not seem to be the prevalent cultural norm. It wasn't uncommon for the friends of Sandy's children to be restricted from all sweets and other treats. Their houses were sugar-free, no chips or salty snacks, and soda was certainly forbidden. When these kids would come to visit Sandy's, if there were any of those foods available, the kids would gorge. Otherwise normal, "healthy living" seemed more like training these children for eating disorders. Sandy took this as a lesson and devised an experiment: She bought a big cookie jar, which she always kept full of some kind of treat and open for business. At first it emptied fast, but soon enough it lost its glamour. Sure, everyone has a cookie now and again, but with the unmonitored open-jar policy, Sandy found herself throwing away stale food more often than finding it bare.

Sandy has much more difficulty with food than her children do—they were not raised to have the same issues. She has improved and is not as obsessed as she used to be, but it's a continuing struggle. She still has a difficult time eating fruit. As a child when the thin ones were permitted ice cream or brownies, she was offered nature's alternative. She "didn't need" treats, she was told. Though, perhaps she did. The more times an eight year old is told an apple is as good as a cookie, the less that apple looks good. Programming to be dysfunctional is highly effective.

It became interesting rather than troublesome to watch as the children matured. Sandy's daughter grew into a womanly size 18 or 20. They work together in a knitting store and her daughter is an expert at recalculating patterns for herself and others so that the knit garments fit perfectly to their size and shape. Sandy watches in wonder and even envy as her daughter does this without the slightest self-consciousness, hesitation, or judgment. Sandy's daughter simply wasn't taught to hate herself or others for who they are. Sandy remembers being young and the disdain from her grandmother when patterns needed adjustment, and the humiliation it caused. Her daughter experiences none of that. Sandy watches her own child in awe.

Her son, who had been growing sideways for years, it seemed out of the blue, used that weight to become tall. At age thirteen, he started his ascent to six foot two inches and didn't gain another pound. He's not a skinny young man, but he's big and strong and doesn't give a second thought to his size or weight.

Now like a team, when they attend family functions, if someone mentions weight Sandy's clan speaks up. Graciously, but in no uncertain terms. They all lovingly express that people are perfect exactly the way they are, and believe it. Sandy finds that she genuinely appreciates all types of bodies now; she says it's as if her eyesight has changed. Her children couldn't imagine it any other way. Her eldest boy has a preference for softer women. That does not surprise Sandy, but what is surprising to her is that it makes her proud.

Sandy notices the joy in people's faces when her children appreciate them for who they are. When a sweater fits perfectly because her daughter has resized the pattern, or her son loves a woman who might by others be condemned as fat, it not only gives her a sense of satisfaction in them, but she also knows that she has been a good mother. Part of a continuous function.

15

SPILLING OVER THE SIDES

Lynn's parents lived through the Great Depression. As such, it might make sense that being able to fatten up your kids would instill a sense of pride, but that just wasn't the case here. As Lynn explains it from her family's perspective, "There's fat—and then there's fat. We didn't have a rosy glow kind of fat; it was a spilling over the sides kind of fat." And that, apparently, was nothing to be proud of.

Lynn is now fifty (plus a little) years old, born in 1962. She was fat from the day she entered the world—and close to 400 pounds now. Her mother had seven children, though one died in infancy. The last three got bigger as she went along, and Lynn was the biggest baby she had. The first four babies came pretty close together, when her mama and daddy were young. Three girls and boy. Then her brother, eight years later, and Lynn nine. Lynn was so much younger than her siblings that she had a niece and nephew before she was even born. So needless to say, most of her siblings were long gone from the house while Lynn was growing up. She and her younger brother remained. He was thin, she was not. Actually, four out of the six children had serious weight issues during their lives, though for some reason, it was not until Lynn that her mother began to question the cause.

At six or seven, Lynn was taken by her mother to the pediatrician to see if she had a thyroid condition. Perhaps that was a fad at the time, because her mother also had three overweight adult children, and there was no particular logic in thinking Lynn was singularly ill. Lynn believes her mother was hoping for a magic bullet—she had enough fat children for her liking. There was no thyroid condition, but there was asthma. Unfortunately, that pediatrician didn't diagnose the asthma, and Lynn lived with it unknowingly until she self-diagnosed as an adult. The asthma made running and playing difficult. Because it was undiagnosed, people thought she was just lazy.

The siblings who were big, Lynn says, all have emotional issues stemming from it. Her mama was born in 1918 and daddy in 1916, with her eldest sister being born in 1939. They all lived through the Depression, so there were residual effects from those years of worry that carried on through Lynn's upbringing. Lynn has a terrible fear of lacking. Her parents always managed to feed the kids, and feed them well, but if ever there was some leftover food, say put away to save for later, someone would snatch it up long before the rightful owner. There was always this pervasive vague sense that there might not ever be more. Consequently, Lynn, and her siblings as well, didn't save much food for later, which may well have contributed to their fat.

But sensitivity to culturally reinforced behavior was not high on the agenda in Lynn's family. While she did experience some bullying in school, what she received from family members was much worse. Her mama's family was notorious for their "picking," as in, "don't take it so hard, I'm just picking on you." Lynn's attitude about this picking was not so casual, and in retrospect, she views it as verbal and emotional abuse. Her uncle, for instance, was a particularly loathsome picker. He used to enjoy leaving family gatherings by telling Lynn, "Next time I see ya, I hope there is less of you to see." To add insult to injury, no one ever stepped in to stop it. Of course, they were afraid the radar would be turned toward them, but that justification didn't make it any easier for Lynn.

Lynn was put on diets repeatedly, usually tagging along with her mother. Whenever her mama would go on a diet, Lynn was required to join in. She grew up eating a lot of cottage cheese, of which she is still not a fan. Nothing really worked, though. Lynn says, "I have a serious appetite, and I've also got a problem. The trigger that tells you that you are full, that supposedly tells you when to stop eating, I don't have that. I recognize it sometimes now, but not often."

There is a genetic condition, Prader-Willi syndrome, that prevents a person from feeling full, and in fact leaves a person feeling starving all the time. Lynn does not have that. But it isn't uncommon for people with a history of disordered eating, including from dieting, to have difficulty recognizing fullness. In fact, recognizing fullness and hunger is central to treatment for disordered eating.

Lynn's mother was not morbidly obese, but she was quite large. "She was more like comfortably heavy—it felt good when you hugged her. And she could work up a huge sweat out in the garden; she had a lot of energy. She was overweight but it didn't stop her from doing anything." Nonetheless, she was perpetually on diets. Lynn's father, on the other hand, was bone thin. Sadly, Lynn's mother died when Lynn was just ten, and that left Lynn and her dad alone together for the rest of her childhood, as the others had all moved out.

Lynn's father was an emotionally withdrawn man. He would offer an occasional pat on the back, but neither Lynn nor her siblings recall him ever saying he loved them. They were Depression-age parents, and Lynn says that means there wasn't much touchy-feely stuff going on. "There weren't a lot of hugs, and we definitely didn't kiss our parents; that was just wrong." Lynn's relationship with food became even more confused when her mother passed. Her father had no idea how to raise a girl alone, much less a fat girl who had lost her mother.

One summer, Daddy bought a freezer full of meat that was supposed to last all winter long. I just got it in my head that we had steak in the freezer, and I was on my own that summer, so I would have a steak sandwich for lunch every day. A year's worth of meat lasted three months. Daddy got upset; I know he got upset about stuff like that, but he didn't know how to handle it. He was just detached. I remember one summer before Mama passed, when I was seven, we went to the beach, and I watched my daddy swim in the ocean. I thought, 'I wish I knew how to do that,' but he never taught me. We never did anything together. Those lines were never crossed.

So whatever dysfunction started before Lynn's mother had passed away continued, and became worse. That, coupled with having a genetic predisposition that her father did not share, made them even more foreign to each other. Neither one of them had the slightest idea what to do.

Lynn is certain at least one of her older sisters was also put on a diet by their mother. By the time Lynn was born, her older sisters were teenagers, and their mama was always reading some new diet magazine, which they would scour for the latest fad to try. When their mother died, Lynn's sisters tried to take over the diet programming for Lynn. She was taken to her first Weight Watchers meeting at the age of thirteen by one of her sisters. And every new year, there would be a group resolution. Lynn still does that today. All the fat siblings tried various diets, with Lynn frequently tagging along. Weight Watchers, Taking Off Pounds Sensibly, fasts. There was always a diet for Lynn when her siblings were involved. At home with her father, though, there was no diet food. He was a rail. He did attempt to help with the Weight Watchers menu as best he could, fixing liver once a week, as prescribed by the Weight Watchers bible. He liked liver, though, so it worked out.

When Lynn was very young and her mother included Lynn in any slimming plan, it was never with anger toward Lynn. She didn't project to Lynn that being fat was a result of weakness or lack of moral fortitude. However, one day Lynn returned from school and her mama asked what the cafeteria had served for lunch. Lynn, for whatever reason, said no lunch had been available because the cafeteria burned down. Mama was livid about the lying. Lynn's sister came to the rescue, with a peculiar conclusion that Lynn was just hungry and wanted a snack—but lacked the creativity for a better plan. So there were mixed messages. Lynn believes her mother's fixation with putting her on diets came from a place of love. The visits to the doctors did as well, though they never particularly made sense given the family history. Her mother was never cruel, but the message was still clear: Fat really wasn't acceptable.

On the other side of the fence, some of Lynn's siblings are certain their father was angry about his fat children, and that he was ashamed. That may have been true, or to him, it was as if aliens landed in his living room; his large children were completely foreign to his ultra-slim experiences. He wished they were thin, as did their mother, but any notion of how to make that come about was a mystery to him. Not that Mama was successful either, but at least she could conceive of a plan. So for their father, paralysis turned to resentment, and shame. That was very hurtful to Lynn. Being fat was enough, without also believing her father was ashamed of her. As if her parents' dismay wasn't sufficient, she too was frustrated beyond comprehension. Many tears have been shed over her lifetime as a result of both the aggravation and humiliation of being fat.

Briefly, while in her twenties, Lynn did lose a considerable amount of weight. Her father was very proud. He would say, "Well, you're able to buy your clothes off the rack now, aren't ya?" That was high praise, certainly intended as a compliment. Lynn, too, enjoyed the idea she could buy clothes off the rack, but that being her father's sense of pride broke her heart. There was no way she knew to communicate this to him, or even process it in her mind. Her parents were born in a different time. They did not engage in deep and meaningful conversation, and even if Lynn wanted to talk these things through, there were no resources. Perhaps there was counseling somewhere in the small town in which she lived, but if there was, no one discussed it. The church and Weight Watchers meetings were as close to a therapeutic environment as it got, and secrets spread like wild fire. God forbid the town should learn about such private matters—which they would, as they made it their mission.

Lynn isn't certain why, at the time, her parents thought the children's weight was a problem. There were no illnesses to blame on weight and there wasn't the frenzied panic there is today, nor the harsh blame. There were, however, stereotypes and standards of beauty. Lynn's parents would see other people's children, thin and pretty, and then their mama couldn't buy her kids the most adorable clothes. When Lynn got older, she was difficult to fit in the fashion of the day. She wanted blue jeans. This was after her mama had died. Her father sent Lynn shopping with her aunt. While Lynn told her aunt she wanted blue jeans, they returned with a sky-blue pants suit. "It's blue, it fits, be happy!"

Lynn suspects having a fat kid does make life details more complex, but she also suspects the overriding conflict was with what Lynn's parents' imagined other people were saying. Though Lynn is not aware of any hurtful or even negative gossip, she guesses there was a perception, or her parents imagined a perception, that the children, and worse, the parents, were lazy. And maybe, in a way, they were—not exactly lazy, perhaps, but disconnected—all the adults in their lives were. When Lynn was taken to the doctor for her theoretical thyroid problem, she was not checked for asthma, despite her trouble breathing. Yet Lynn lived in a home filled with secondhand smoke. It was a different time, certainly, but not all of the factors that might impact Lynn's ability to run and play were considered. For that matter, they still generally aren't. Fat still means lazy, and gluttonous, to most. Actually, now more than ever, other factors are considered suspect offhand.

At any rate, it was important to Lynn's parents that neither they nor their children appeared to be lazy. To them lazy meant slovenly, and slovenly meant poor, and poor meant desperate. "We weren't white trash, but we weren't that far from it." Both of her parents worked. Her mother in a hospital as a nurses' aide, and her father owned a tiny one-room market, which he bankrupted. Her father, kind at heart in such matters, offered credit to anyone, and it was his downfall. After Lynn was born, he drove a bread truck.

They attended the most prestigious church in town, as did any family trying to appear up-and-coming. Though her mama would never admit to her pride, she very much wanted to make a good impression. Lynn heard rumor there were people who looked down upon them at their church, but she didn't witness any actual evidence. Lynn suspects that the truth, no matter what her mother feared and imagined, was that most people didn't bother to give them any consideration, one way or another. "And if they did, it shouldn't have mattered. But it did. You'd think that people who lived through the Depression would be proud to fatten up the children, but there is fat, and then there is really fat. Maybe they thought we were just too fat."

Lynn's parents clearly felt some amount of shame about their fat children, but it is not clear if they felt any guilt. That may have been an honor reserved for Lynn's siblings. It wasn't that long ago that Lynn's eldest sister revealed that she took the blame for Lynn's weight, believing that her own fatness was somehow the cause of the fatness in the younger ones. By allowing herself to be fat, she perhaps projected a sense that fat was acceptable, and in her lack of becoming thin, she demonstrated a poor dieting work ethic. Lynn's sister felt she was a poor role model, and even inadvertently, an advocate of overweight. Lynn did not accept the blame of her sister, because she was too busy blaming herself. "You didn't hold up the fork to my mouth; I did that myself." There are times when Lynn wishes she could stop eating altogether—never having to eat again. It would be easier to have self-control if there is nothing at all to prime the pump of temptation. Of course, Lynn didn't invent this idea for a weight-loss method; it is the heart and soul of anorexia.

So both Lynn and her sister feel as though they are the villains when it comes to Lynn's fat body, but not the only ones. "There were three others who were fat, and I know that Mama was the one that fed us. Maybe it was a Depression thing, but if we said we wanted more she never said no, that I can remember." But the blame is circular. In the next breath, Lynn mentions the fork she put to her mouth, again. The reason for the fat is confusing to Lynn. Or worse. Mystifying. Confounding. Infuriating. Both logical and completely absurd. The fat is her fault, it is the fault of others, and it's the fault of no one. Whoever the culprit, it is as if she has had a knife plunged in the center of her back, and she is unable to reach it for removal no matter how she contorts herself. That knife, and the effort to remove it, are her life's work. Or in a different analogy, Lynn is Sisyphus and her fat is the boulder.

In nearly every fat child's life, there is bound to be an episode or dozen that haunts for years into the future. When Lynn was eleven or twelve, she had a girlfriend who was going through a personal trauma. This friend would call Lynn each night and talk her ear off for hours, seeking support and consolation, which Lynn would generously provide. These armchair therapy sessions went on for months—until the girl's birthday rolled around. She planned a party in which all the guests were to ride on a horse, as was quite fashionable at the time. Lynn wasn't invited. Apparently the girl's family feared Lynn would be too heavy for the horse's back. In truth, that reason is only speculation on Lynn's part, and what she continues to believe to this day. It seems she never asked and they never told. Now, whether a horse would be too frail to carry the weight of almost any eleven-year-old is worth a ponder, and Lynn may have been quite fat, but too fat for a horse? Unlikely. But perception isn't always reality. Among the other memories that haunt her include that she, of course, was always picked last for teams. With the exception of the game Red Rover.

There she was a ringer, the only girl who could barrel though the wall of boys when called to come over.

Though Lynn's eldest sister had the most to say about the weight of her siblings, she is not the only one, besides Lynn, who seemed emotionally affected. Lynn is not certain what exactly prompted it, but she suspects some of her brothers and sisters have eating disorders. She has been at various times a closet eater, and prone to episodes of bingeing as well. This is not at all uncommon for dieters, particularly ones with a lifelong habit. However, there may be other reasons as well. Being so much younger than her siblings, she was a bit of a novelty to their friends—sort of a mascot. When out joyriding, they would bring her along to cruise, and invariably end up at various fast-food joints. There, the local football players would carry Lynn around, and the other teenagers would amuse themselves by feeding her—sort of like she was their pet goat. This was a great deal of fun for Lynn, and an excellent way to learn that attention, whether positive or otherwise, was linked with food. This may have exacerbated matters, but the truth is, Lynn did not become fat from these episodes or any other trip to the burgeoning fast-food eateries. It started long before that.

Lynn can come up with this or that explanation. For instance, her mother made Southern foods, always cooked with fatback and a lot of salt. In fact, her mother salted everything—she never ate a piece of fruit or a vegetable without salt. Lynn did too, at the time, though no longer. But these sorts of things are typical enough, particularly while Lynn was growing up. There were certainly plenty of Southern-food eaters in the 1960s and '70s who did not become large. And today, there is a resurgence of cooking with lard, those who think that natural fat is healthier than processed fats, even olive oil. Whether it is or isn't, considering the amount of time during her childhood Lynn was eating cottage cheese rather than fried chicken, Sunday dinners were not the cause of her young obesity, either.

There is much discussion of the role of genetics in weight, and indisputable scientific correlation. Despite that, Lynn isn't one of those people who blame their family lineage. With so many years of being programmed to believe she is the cause of her body size, and shamefully so, it is difficult for her to internalize the idea that fat ran in the family due to genes, and not gluttony.

> It never occurred to me that it was something genetic, that there were just fat people. Even saying it now, it's like, what is that, genetic fat? It can't be a real thing. I honestly don't know. Oh my gosh, I guess it could be that way, but honestly, no, it was something bad, that could be controlled. Thinking about it now, it's kind of mind-blowing. We figured we were fat because we were eating too much. I guess that's why we all thought it was our fault. Our mom didn't do anything all that different, that we should be fat and not other people. She cooked Southern cooking, but there were a lot of thin kids who ate Southern cooking. I don't know if my mother thought it was her fault. My older sister did. She thought that she was a bad example, that she was fat and didn't work hard enough, and set a bad example for us. But no one dieted more than she did, no one worked harder.

Although she started dieting with her mother at a very young age, Lynn put on most of her weight after her mama died, when Lynn was in her early teens. "On Saturdays, I would eat nonstop. I would describe it as if I woke up with a chicken leg in each hand. I ate all day. Then all of a sudden, it was as if I came to. I guess that was really good binge eating going on. It was a comfort, after losing Mama at such a young age. Eating still offers me comfort sometimes, but not as much."

Lynn was a lonely child; she spent quite a bit of time alone, and despite her large family, there was a sense of loneliness about many of them. "All of us were shy. It was difficult making friends. Loneliness was an issue for a lot of us. It still is for me. There is sadness eating, and stress eating. We were swallowing food to try to desensitize ourselves." So there was genetics, and food, and emotions, and then genetics, and food, and emotions again. Still, half the family was fat, and half was not.

> One thing I can remember is supposed friends would clip your Achilles' heel when you were least expecting it. There was a girl I can remember that signed one of my yearbooks. After telling me to have a wonderful summer and all that stuff, she signed it off with "So nice going to school with ya, fatty. Just kidding, ha ha." That's something that's going to live with you forever.

So often, fat people do exactly the same things thin people do, but fat people get punished for it—in two ways. First we get fat, and then people tell us we're lazy, gluttonous, slobs for being fat.

At fifty, Lynn is a newlywed. He is wonderful man who loves Lynn dearly, and she him. But he is concerned for her health.

> He says that's why he wants me to lose weight. But because of all the baggage I have, I feel like I am being chastised or punished. He loves me no matter what, but just the fact that he mentions it, it opens up way too many closets full of skeletons. I know he doesn't mean to hurt my feelings, but once you've been a fat kid, everything hurts your feelings. I'm so tired of letting people down. Maybe I'll tell him it's just my genetics and to leave me alone, except deep down I still think it's my fault. I am still constantly looking for the perfect diet, if you happen to know one.

16

IF AT FIRST YOU DON'T SUCCEED, GIVE UP!

As far back as Betsy can recall, she remembers her body being larger than the bodies of other kids. Her parent's memories go back even farther. Though her mom's side of the family was thin, that was not the case with her father's. He had always been overweight, as had most of his relatives. Betsy looked like her dad's kin, and he was conscious of Betsy's weight before Betsy even understood what being weight-conscious meant.

Betsy was primarily raised by her mother. Her parents divorced, and soon after her dad was remarried. In between wives, her father went on a strict diet and exercise regime. He became much thinner and has since made the gym his second home. He also became even more aware of Betsy's size and shape. It made for an interesting dynamic for Betsy, growing up. While she felt more emotionally connected to her mother's side of the family, she looked like she belonged to her dad's—well, except her own father, when he stopped looking like he was related to himself. Despite or perhaps because of his relatives, her father openly expressed his thoughts on Betsy's body, though it was her mother who dealt with the ramifications from day to day. Her mother's way to deal was primarily by focusing on other things—like education and self-esteem. She didn't make Betsy's body a central theme. But, the world being the world, by fourth or fifth grade there was no way to distract Betsy from her own fat. At that point, it was no longer just Mom against Dad. It was also Betsy against the world.

By nine years old, all the girls were acutely aware of fat and spent a great deal of time thinking and talking about it. Education and self-esteem were no match for thin thighs. Betsy felt she was fatter than her peers, and perhaps she was. But regardless of her size, her perception of her looks, as compared to others, was what really mattered. Rumor had it that one of the girls had gone on a diet. That was an exciting event. Not only did Betsy think the girl looked amazing, but even more important, so did her friends. Betsy wanted those kinds of accolades and that kind of acceptance, too, so she wanted to diet. Thus, in the sixth grade, Betsy went on her first official diet. Her mother dieted with her out of solidarity. Betsy did lose some weight, but immediately thereafter her best friend from out of town came to visit and dieting gave way to celebrating. Betsy gained the weight back, plus more. That was her first real diet, and her first real post-diet weight gain. It wouldn't be her last.

Afterward, Betsy became very depressed. And rather than admiration and enthusiasm from her classmates, she was bullied and shunned. It was certainly not the desired outcome of the dieting process. In fact, Betsy was so traumatized by the whole debacle she was unable to finish her eighth grade year in school. Emotionally, she was done. Betsy got home-schooled to complete those middle years and proudly graduated eighth grade from her kitchen. For the ninth grade, she enrolled in a private school, where it was hoped she would be appreciated more, and bullied less. There was, in fact, more of an emphasis on schoolwork at the new place, and though she didn't exactly fit in, she managed to get through, graduating early.

Betsy went right on to college, where she expected the world to be a completely different place—full of free thinkers and tolerance. Whether it was or wasn't, Betsy was still the same person. On her own, she gained a great deal of weight. Weight, and the

idea that her body was encased in too much of it, was an integral
part of her self-image. Fat was who she was, and recognizing that
made her feel hopeless. Betsy began to feel a sense of doom about
her entire life. With each new rite of passage, which she anticipated would make things better, it got worse. And she got fatter. Or,
she got fatter with each new rite of passage, and things got worse.
Either way, she was fat, and there seemed no way out of the trap.

Her premonition that she was destined for an angst-filled life
began to clarify when she realized she wanted to experience romance. It seemed as though people enjoyed her company, appreciated her personality, liked her as a human being, but when it came
to romance, she was the girl holding up the wall at the dance.
That one aspect of her perceived reality felt like a disavowal of
her as a full person. Along with that sense of alienation came
shame and disappointment.

Betsy had been raised with immense pressure to be successful
as a professional. She was informed she was given opportunities
her parents didn't have, and it was her responsibility to exploit
them. This caused more conflict. Successful professional women
didn't look as she did; she knew that. How could a woman with
her appearance succeed? Though she wasn't interested in business or law, if she had been, it would have been moot. Those
types of women are thin. They must be; they wear form-fitting
suits. Of course, athletics wasn't in her future—those outfits were
even more revealing. She did join the swim team in her freshman
year of college, but only under duress, as a sport was a require-
ment. Her team members were not exactly supportive—and she
overheard a young child at the pool asking his father why someone like her even bothered. The father responded respectfully; he
wasn't overtly teaching his son to judge. But if a seven year old
inherently knew Betsy as a swimmer was absurd, surely everyone
else did as well—they merely had more grace in public.

At least in part because of how she perceived her place in the
world, Betsy gravitated toward the social sciences—women's
studies in particular. It was a safe place for a fat girl. Nearly a

cliché. But it worked well for her; she felt accepted. She didn't stick out in women's studies, because all the women stuck out. Being among her own kind, outcasts, helped to raise Betsy's consciousness about feminist issues, and particularly body image as a feminist issue. This changed her life in many ways. She began to have a drive to help other people, women younger than she, to recognize that all those experiences, feelings of alienation, were not a result of an inherit flaw, but stemmed from something much larger and more powerful than the person: societal ideals. She also came to the realization that she had possessed a limited, even biased, notion of what professional women are supposed to look like, and overall, which bodies are allowed to fit in which spaces.

Shaping those perspectives, she learned, was in large part the media. Betsy had been a voracious MTV watcher in middle school—and as she considered what she watched, she realized it was built to warp perceptions of what women should, or could, be. She remembers her mother quipping that Betsy was such an accomplished arguer, she might consider becoming a lawyer or politician. Quip as it might have been, there had been politicians in the family, so it wasn't far-fetched. But that career path never seemed feasible to Betsy, she didn't have the body for the job. She thought it best to pursue endeavors that kept her from the public eye, that allowed her to hide her shame. That was more suited to a fat woman.

Betsy's mother never wished for her daughter to escape the outside world; that was not the message she tried to impart. But Betsy's peers and the media were more convincing than a mother. They seemed so much more objective, not clouded by blind motherly love. Betsy's epiphany that she was not the right size for acceptance in the public realm made her very unhappy—and even worse, it supported the notion that she was hopelessly doomed. Her mother's attempts to acknowledge Betsy's feelings seemed to validate them. Not her mother's intentions, of course, but for Betsy it was all murky. It seemed like an endless loop of words and images informing her she belonged behind closed doors.

Her father had a different approach; he tried to be objective about her body and frame his concerns around health. Undisputed, he believed, fat was unhealthy, and the rest was of no great import. His attitude resulted in some positive interactions. He bought Betsy a bike and took her along for walks. This helped Betsy to realize her body was more powerful and capable than she had thought. But it didn't erase the sense of doom—if she didn't lose weight, her whole life would be wrong, and short. She would be sick. Have a heart attack. Live with a sense of impending and inevitable disaster. Her father's focus on health, and concern for health, presented moments of light, but mostly resulted in an underlying and constant sense of panic.

During one particular incident, Betsy joined her father on a morning run, though she was on her bike, and he was running in a group of four men. When they returned, Betsy was dizzy and tired. The excursion was too much for her, and that was humiliating, which wasn't helped by that fact that her father seemed embarrassed and disappointed by her performance. He never took her on one of his runs again. He also saw it as a sign that Betsy would never lose weight. She would always be fat and always be a failure. Her destiny determined at the age of ten.

Years later, Betsy and her father set out on a four-mile hike together. It wasn't an easy hike and about every ten minutes her dad would check in. "I don't want you to have a heart attack. Don't fall. I don't want you to go to the hospital. And, I can't carry you out." That sort of thing. Betsy was no longer ten and by this time Betsy knew her body. Besides, the hike was her idea, and she wasn't the slightest bit concerned something tragic would occur. What did irritate Betsy was her father's lack of faith in her assessment of her capabilities. It was evident she was not an individual person to him, just a statistic. In fact, Betsy's father had never experienced a connection between fat and ill health in his own life—not with family or friends. He just accepted it as gospel. Betsy thinks his perceptions may be wrapped up in some prejudice, against his own upbringing. He grew up poor, and the women were, and still are, fat. He was the first one in the line to attend college and be a success. He was also the first to lose weight. The assumptions made about poverty and obesity, and wealth and thinness, are common enough. He never stated any of this out loud, but Betsy sees the signs.

Betsy's father was fat when he met her mom. His fatness seemed to be part of his identity as a Midwestern farmer. Those boys are husky. But he got his master's degree in agricultural science, and although he was never a suit-and-tie kind of guy, he became more of a businessman, and his sense of himself seemed to change. He came from hardworking and hearty stock. They were fat, but not necessarily obese, Betsy says. These were capable people. They never talked about weight, other than to congratulate Betsy's dad when he lost it. To Betsy, the idea of being fat and capable on a farm did not translate to being fat and capable in a courtroom. There were certain people who could pull off being fat, and others who couldn't.

Although her father never encouraged her to diet, exactly, he was very vocal about food, and food choices. Dinners included a lot of instruction on proper eating habits. Not too many carbs, no butter on the vegetables. He didn't hesitate to inform her if she was engaging in a behavior he found irresponsible. Betsy found herself to be more self-regulating around her father, more so than when she wasn't with him, and she resented that. For one thing, she was a young woman trying to foster a sense of independence, and it was irritating having her father tell her what to do. But perhaps more important, and more significant long term, it inhibited Betsy from having a good sense of her own body's needs. It also confused her relationship to food. Though she never had a clinical eating disorder, she did experience a disconnect that she worked to resolve for many years.

To say her father, or for that matter other family members, didn't encourage Betsy to diet isn't exactly true. They didn't demand it, but they did find ways to make it seem palatable. Her father paid for Nutrisystem. And, her grandmother offered her twenty dollars for every pound she lost. This did not sit well with Betsy. But at the time she was living in the same town with these people, and it was difficult to escape their thoughtful support, or critical judgment, depending on how you perceive it. Betsy recalls driving back from a county fair once; she was in the backseat while her grandmother and aunt were in the front. The two were having a grand old time laughing at some fat woman they had seen. They were like "mean girls" and Betsy the fat nerd behind them, forced to accept the ridicule on someone else's behalf in silence, or perhaps have it turned on her. She was only in high school at the time and living that experience daily in another world. She was bullied at school, and bullied secondhand in the backseat of the family car. There was no escaping it, and nowhere she fit in.

The truth is, though, Betsy was different, although not in the ways some might imagine. This only made her frustration and alienation stronger. When she went on that first diet with her mother, and then gained the weight back, it was an unusual time. Dieting was not typical for her and neither was all of the celebrating that came after, with the visiting of old friends. In the usual course of events, Betsy ate normally, that is to say well—which perhaps wasn't normal at all. Both of her parents were cognizant to prepare healthy foods, complete, nutritious meals. In fact, Betsy would be shocked when she visited a thin friend's home and there would be sugar cereals and candy bars on the shelves for the taking, as if that were normal. These people might grab a bite for dinner, whatever was around; they even ate fast-food. That was unheard of in Betsy's house. Her parents taught her to love whole grains and fresh vegetables. She didn't necessarily develop that love as a child, but she did eventually, and it never made sense that out of all these people she knew, she was the fat one. It seemed so unjust. To add insult to injury, she was a health nut, but she got accused of the behavior of her thin friends. It seemed obvious to the world that she was the one who ate crap. And who would believe her if she told them otherwise?

Betsy has given a great deal of thought to why she was fat, when her peers were not. First there is genetics, but she doesn't blame that entirely. Though she recognizes when people do blame genetics they often get shut down. No one seems to believe it's just genetics, and if you are a fat person and claim it is in your genes, you are branded a liar. So whether true or false, Betsy looks to environmental factors too.

> I think as with any natural or biological thing there are environmental factors, and I definitely think it was very hard for me to have a straightforward relationship with my own body. I didn't have a good sense of how I felt, or when eating a particular thing made me feel better or worse. I was so used to feeling bad about my body all the time that those signals didn't get sent. I've spent a lot of time trying to listen more to them, not worrying about what I look like, but what feels good. When I was younger, I had the sense that there was an ideal body and if I didn't reach the ideal, I failed, and if I was going to fail, there was no point in even trying. Now I am much more realistic. I can feel healthier or less healthy, and feeling healthier is better. But I am never going to look like Super Model X, nor should I really want to. It's impossible with my genetics.
>
> I was less likely to want to eat healthy and exercise when I was younger because I felt like there was no point. I was not going to get the result I idealized, so I became stuck. I was unable to pay attention to my body. Between the ages of eight and twenty-five, things got really complicated for me, I couldn't think for myself, there was all this outside interference. When I wasn't at home, when I had mobility, I ate junk food, a lot of fast-food. I couldn't sense how it made me feel. I just knew I felt trapped and was breaking free. Also, other kids ate junk food too. I wasn't doing anything all that different from them, and

that was frustrating. We did the same things with different results. It felt like a personal failing, like it was my fault.

That sense wasn't helped by incidents like the bike-riding episode. In retrospect, Betsy realizes she was just a little kid, maybe ten years old. The ride was too much at her age and she had neglected to bring water. She didn't become unwell because she was fat or lazy; she was dehydrated. Yet no one considered that, and her father's seeming disappointment left Betsy feeling like a failure. She was ashamed as a result of being compared to her father. They all, Betsy included, seemed to have the idea a young and healthy child should have more energy than a grown man. And maybe in some cases this is true. But this was her first excursion and he did the route every day. Should a ten-year-old girl have the stamina of a youthful and fit adult male, and additionally need no hydration? The answer doesn't matter because he never took her again. That Betsy was unable to identify her body's cues was not just because she was fat, genetically or otherwise. It was environmental too— learned because that was what she was taught.

When Betsy reflects on it now, what she finds most troubling, and also bizarre, is how because of her fatness, she was discouraged from doing the things that people believed supported thinness. She experienced this with her father, but also in school, with her peers, and other members of the family: Since she wasn't particularly athletic, athletics wasn't the sort of thing she should be doing in public. She was literally discouraged. No one seemed to think she should be out there, whether it be for health or fun. Her lack of innate ability meant she should be relegated to the corner. Thus, she was damned if she did and damned if she didn't. Mocked as a fat kid who wasn't good at sports, and mocked if she attempted to improve.

At the time, this attitude brought Betsy a sense of relief. It was much more comfortable to slink away. It was embarrassing enough to be who she was, much less be who she was while running, jumping, and jiggling. But by the time she was a teenager, she began to recognize the irony, and was not pleased. "I think as I got a little older, even by middle school, and certainly by high school, I started to notice the contradiction in the way people talked about body image and health, and expectations about behavior." It wasn't only about exercise that Betsy experienced peculiar perceptions, not necessarily based on best judgment, or even reality.

> It's been interesting, because I lost so much weight at one point. My parents and my family were really excited about me losing the weight. Pretty much everybody I came in contact with was excited about it. I felt like, now I'm off the hook, they're not going to bother me about this anymore because I am doing something that is pleasing to them. It's like I proved to them I was aware about my health in a way that wasn't apparent to them before. Then I gained a lot of the weight back. Did I somehow forget what I became aware of?
>
> Then I recently bought a bike and I was trying to get back into it after eighteen years. The first time I rode it I had a huge anxiety attack. I talked to my stepmom about it, thinking she's a pretty sympathetic and understanding person, and her response was to give me a big lecture about my health and how I just needed to suck it up and do it. This was right after I had gone on that hike with my dad, where I was fine, but he didn't think I should do it because I would drop dead on the spot.
>
> After that, I called them up and told them that I didn't want to talk about my weight anymore, period. "It's my body, it's my decision, what I chose to do or not do is my business. I don't want to have this conversation with you again." So that's where it stands now; I don't really want their opinion about my body or its size. With my mom, I still talk to her about it, but honestly, there isn't that much of a conversation to have.

Betsy had been fighting judgment for so long, on so many fronts, that there is really only so much a person can take. In middle school when she became terribly depressed and decided she had to leave, she made a list of all the kids who had bullied her. Then all the kids who had been sort of complacent and just let the bullying happen before their eyes, doing nothing. And finally the kids who defended her, were true friends, or at the very least stayed away from the abusive incidents. The majority of the school was in the first two lists. Her mom sent the lists to the school, telling them specifically who was responsible. "These people are bullying my daughter. Are you going to do anything about it?" The school responded there was nothing they could do. Nothing.

This is how activists are made, if they aren't beaten down too far.

In theory, Betsy supports some of the newer messages to children about health, and they are certainly better than focusing on weight.

But it's often difficult for anyone, let alone children, to make the distinction. I feel like I got so much outside information, other people's opinions about my own body, that it was really hard for me to develop my own sense of myself. It took me ten years of adult life to feel that I am comfortable in my skin most of the time. It was all the messages, not just the negative ones, but also the more positive ones, about health choices. I had a strong feeling for a very long time that it didn't matter how healthy my choices were, if I didn't look a certain way, people were going to perceive me as unhealthy. I don't think I have seen any programs aimed at youth that really address differences, especially body differences—having a standard or an idea that starts wherever the kid is and helps them improve from where they are, rather than comparing them to normal. These kids are always the outliers, and if you are an outlier there is an implication there is something wrong with you.

I remember being in gym in sixth or seventh grade and we were doing the statewide physical fitness testing. We were doing push-ups and had to call out the number we reached. I yelled out fifteen and the gym teacher stopped the procession and looked perplexed. He didn't believe someone like me could do fifteen push-ups. And I was like, "Of course I can do that many; I'm really strong, duh." But I felt singled out, and the whole program was meant to be encouraging—at least it was supposed to be. It was supposed to get kids to want to be more physically active. That certainly wasn't the experience I had. I was different, so I must be bad.

And that certainly didn't help Betsy become more physically active. How could anyone in her right mind believe that it would?

In the end, it seems Betsy was right to find a safe place to grow her mind and career. It afforded her the opportunity to stop the pointless things people encouraged, like dieting, and begin in earnest the things that had been discouraged, like taking good care of her body, despite being fat. Sometimes giving up is the best way to succeed.

17

IT'S NOT THE SIZE
THAT MATTERS

Kate is athletic, happy, healthy, and fat. She has not always been athletic, happy, and healthy, but she has always been fat. At least for as long as she can remember. Not as an infant or toddler, but in preschool, the baby fat lingered, and from there she grew in every direction. It is not insignificant that she grew up as well as out—she was not only the roundest kid, but also the longest, and for her size and stature she was mercilessly teased. After all, she was a big, big girl, so she deserved to be punished. Obviously.

Today Kate is athletic, happy, and healthy because she worked very hard to overcome the problems of her body that other people informed her she had. She did so through therapy, mainly. She was treated for post-traumatic stress disorder. She had been through a war, waged by perception.

Though Kate has had the same body for a long time—in fact, her entire life—she has not always felt a sense of belonging with it. In other words, she had trouble relating to herself. The disconnect started early; she found it difficult to feel ownership of what others seemed to view as merely a human mass. The body somehow seemed otherworldly, and attached to her by pure happenstance. Kate simply wasn't comfortable in her own skin, which made it all the more difficult to care for, much less love it. Even her memories of her body seemed surreal. Her brain had created some kind of barrier between the gray matter and all that was connected. She was a mind inside some ornate, though not attractive packaging. When they built her, they seemed to choose the wrong box. Of course this was not reality as others saw it, but it was her reality, and it did reflect the reality she perceived others saw. One point of confusion plagued Kate for many years: How could such a good brain be responsible for such a bad body? And she did have a good brain. That was a puzzle Kate was not able to solve for a great deal of her life.

Part of the difficulty in putting together all the pieces was the paradox of living in a body that people expected should be different, yet were intolerant of in the act of attempting to change. Kate feared doing anything physical in the presence of others. She dared not run, compete in sports, or be active in general, because she was surely the slowest or most awkward or out of breath. She was humiliated for being who she was and humiliated in her attempts to be different. She was caught between her body and the world.

The same was true when it came to how she felt and what she ate. Her emotions seeded her eating, which seeded her emotions. She was never taught the difference between feeling sad or angry or disappointed or even loathing of herself, and being hungry. Soothing became eating and eating became hating and Kate became unable to do anything but disconnect as a result.

Kate first attempted to be invisible in the second or third grade. She figured the slower she moved the less likely she was to be seen. And she certainly didn't want to be seen, because she looked nothing like those around her. She didn't have their speed or stamina, nor did she have their attire. This was about the time when she became unable to dress in the clothing made for girls her age, and she was forced to wear the fashion skin of an adult. So she was tall and fat and slow and dressed like a grown-up and mistaken for a failure, though very much just a child.

At home the world was disintegrating as quickly as she was disconnecting. Her parents were preoccupied with the degradation of their relationship, which by the time Kate was ten, split in two. And just at that point, Kate's mother was diagnosed with a medical condition. She was found to have type 1 diabetes, even though an adult. Insulin-dependent. Her body had to be monitored, lanced, and injected for it to remain whole.

Kate's mother always had a difficult relationship with weight and food, which she projected onto Kate, whether she realized it or not. And now there were changes that were necessary, not just perceived. Sugars and sweets were forbidden for Kate's mother, and therefore, for Kate. Whenever there was an adjustment made to Kate's mother's intake, so it was to Kate's as well. If Kate's mother dieted, Kate dieted. If Kate's mother restricted, Kate restricted too.

But it was not just the food plan that Kate's mother shared, it was her attitude about being fat. If Kate was perceived to be eating too much or caught snacking when snacking was prohibited, Kate's mother would puff out her cheeks, hold her arms wide to the side, and mimic a gigantic fat thing. Roly-poly. Laden with fat. Shuffling, puffing, putrid, and stuffed. No words were necessary when this was displayed; Kate knew exactly what it meant, and how it felt. It meant, "Don't get more fat," and it felt crushing. The diagnosis was a huge transition in Kate's mother's life, which neither of them had the maturity to handle.

Kate was about eight or nine when her mother began including her in food-restriction regimes. At the time, there was a great deal of snack food in the house, cookies and other treats. Kate experienced many mixed messages at that time. Though she was not to be fat, there were no substantive conversations about food. No explanations. She was taught to clean her plate at dinner regardless of hunger, but there was displeasure if Kate ate the snack food regardless of hunger. Inconsistency was a constant.

Kate doesn't recall if there were specific rules about snacks, but she expected that if she asked the answer would be no. That is when Kate began sneaking and bingeing. Just around the same time her mother was diagnosed. Despite the illness, Kate's mother did not remove the foods that were problematic for a diabetic. It seemed as if the presence of these foods were a test, for everyone. Kate's mother fought to change her own behavior, though not the conditions under which she lived. She still hasn't. Kate was expected to do the same. It was not until many years later during a visit, when Kate was scolded for eating some snack food, that Kate realized her mother was actually talking to herself. By this time Kate had learned to eat only what she actually wanted and not to binge. Her mother, it seemed, had more trouble.

Kate's mother was not fat herself. In fact she was a petite woman. Her diabetes was type 1; she was never accused of acquiring it because of weight. There were times when she was slightly heavier than others, but never what Kate would call fat. She was also a bit of an exercise nut; she taught physical education and aerobics. Now Kate calls her buff mother "super-jacked."

Aside from there being a house full of snacks, the meals Kate's mother prepared were balanced, made from scratch. After the split, food at Kate's father's was less ideal, from a diet-friendly standpoint. There was a regular routine—Chinese food on Tuesdays, pizza on Thursdays, and leftovers for school lunch the next day. But that had little if anything to do with Kate's mother's attitude, which began earlier and was more a reflection of her own issues than Kate's.

There was certainly a history of overweight people in Kate's extended family, but mostly on her father's side. Her dad has always been large and so has his family. In Kate's mother's family there were larger men, but the women were slender and petite. Although Kate's father was a big guy himself, and often talked about his own struggles with weight, he never mentioned Kate's size when she was a child. In fact if she brought it up he would change the subject to himself, wistfully contemplating getting back down to 200 pounds. He discussed his own workouts; he believed exercise was the key. It's not entirely clear, but he seemed to be hesitant to judge her. He would try to relate, apparently expressing he understood the plight of fat, but Kate was never mocked or shamed by her father. Their relationship is better for it. They do on occasion have a heart-to-heart that goes both ways. It's safer now.

When Kate talks of sneaking food as a child, there is a curious implication that it was an inevitability, in fact, a natural progression. If snack food was available, it was to be eaten, but only in secret. Forbidden, unless cloaked in secrecy. Upon reflection, Kate doesn't actually think it is, or should be, an ordinary evolution that a child would steal and binge in private. But in her environment it just made sense. Clearly these foods were there for a purpose, and that purpose wasn't communal enjoyment. The items were most likely there to test resolve, to fall back on when resolve was not enough, as reward, and as punishment.

As so many do, Kate used sneaking and bingeing as self-regulation when she was upset or otherwise had an emotional reaction. She associated those snacks with feeling better, until she ate them, and then she became ashamed. Her mother knew she was pilfering the snacks. For one, Kate would get caught in the act often enough, and also, her mother bought them. When two Oreos are missing, perhaps a little mouse took them. When it's thirteen, that mouse is more likely a rat. Now that Kate buys her own Oreos, she realizes how absurd it was to think half of a bag would go unnoticed, but at twelve years old, perspective on that sort of thing can a bit skewed.

After the first few, it wasn't so much the taste that mattered. After the first few, they don't even really taste that good. Kate says it was the "mouth feel." That was the comfort. She was going for the soothing sensation of touching them with her tongue and chewing them with her teeth. Also, food is associated with feeling cared for, and satisfaction. As a child there are only so many things that can bring about those feelings. Kate may have seen her mother use food the same way, but it is just as likely she stumbled upon the connection early, perhaps at birth.

Kate doesn't remember getting into trouble, precisely, when she would be caught. There is no memory of a specific reaction, scolding, or punishment. Frankly, the shame was enough. Kate punished herself more than her mother could ever punish her. Whether her mother was aware of that, Kate doesn't know.

Kate's relationship with her mother was quite complicated. That is how she views it now, after therapy. Kate perceived her mother as fragile, and believed the responsibility for keeping their world stable fell to herself. She worked very hard as a child to do that. It was a tall order for any young person, but for Kate in particular, as there had been a great deal of chaos and very little stability in her experiences. Tragically, Kate had been molested by her grandfather—her mother's father. She never discussed this with her mother. She is not sure whether or not her mother had been sexually abused as well, but she believes at least one other relative had. Kate cannot claim whether this is specifically tied to her particular coping mechanism but is aware of research that links childhood obesity and sexual abuse. Certainly not all or even most large children have been sexually abused, but there are neurobiological impacts of childhood trauma, and a connection has been found in some.

In Kate's case, she was abused between the ages of three and seven, and her bingeing began at age eight. That is not to say it was a direct link. Other things were going on at this time as well. But she felt as she said, quite disconnected. She felt disconnected in general and when she was eating. Though to her, eating was an attempt to get back in connection with her body. Full, satisfied, safe. She was striving for that. She had difficulty judging when she was full, much less satisfied or safe. But at least eating made Kate feel human. The act of eating. The taste of eating. The sensation of eating. The feelings of eating. It was an attempt to bring herself back to some sense of reality, perhaps lost when she was trau- matized. Kate began treatment for post-traumatic stress disorder much later, to begin to reconnect with her body.

Her parents to this day don't know that Kate was abused, as her grandfather is still alive and her mother is a caretaker for him, and Kate cannot see unsettling that now. When she does tell them, and she will eventually, it will be very difficult for them all, she knows. Kate has modest contact with her grandfather, but only when necessary. Her mother pressured her to develop more of a relationship, for a while, until Kate put an end to it. She suspects her mother suspects. She doesn't think her father has any inkling. Someday.

As an adult, Kate has become a counselor. She perceives several different connections between sexual abuse and obesity or eating disorders. The first and most obvious is behavioral, and is particularly notable in issues like anorexia nervosa. It is about control. Control over one's body and what one does, or does not, put into it. That could also apply in other eating disorders, bingeing and purging, and related compulsive exercising. Then there is self-protection. Some people attempt to use their body size to distance themselves from others. Though none of these connections are true for everyone who was abused, has an eating disorder, or is considered obese. However, Kate relates to these concepts.

For Kate, although she thought she wanted to be thin, she also believes her body size was used as a buffer against the world. While she admired the cute clothing that the other girls wore, she donned oversized and baggy garments to hide within. She longed to date, but feared that anyone might pay her too much attention. She thought that as a fat person, she could avoid sexual relationships, and even emotional connections.

Kate cultivated a persona that put her on the defensive. In the eighth grade she became a vegetarian for the protection of animals. She joined activist groups like Amnesty International and wore Birkenstocks and clogs, T-shirts from left-wing liberal groups, a wardrobe she perceived as the activist's uniform. Though Kate felt she was a very warm person, she was told she was punkish and inaccessible. Being fat, for her, was part of that persona.

Kate had been teased since the fourth or fifth grade, and it continued through junior high school. Not only was she fat, and tall, but she hit puberty young and by that time had already developed breasts. Though specific instances are vague, she remembers it being virtually a continual battle. It was so upsetting she attempted to get her mother to enroll her in private school starting in elementary. That did not happen.

In the eighth grade, prior to high school, Kate had a boyfriend, a young man she had met in a church youth group. They would write each other notes and hold hands watching television after school. Kate broke up with him, thinking she liked another boy better, though he turned out to be her last boyfriend until she was a senior. He is now, and was then, gay, but they were a perfect cover for each other, as neither had any inclination toward initiating sex. When Kate did finally agree to sexual activity, she was in college, and it was always in the dark, as covered as possible, and most flatteringly positioned.

Although she was included in whatever meal plan her mother was into at the time, mostly by default, Kate wasn't a big dieter when she was young. She tried LA Weight Loss in high school and would periodically start an exercise regime, which would consist of gearing up with baggy sweatpants, an oversized T-shirt, and her Sport Discman, and going outside for a two-block sprint, after which she got tired and went home. There was frequently something in the works to begin at a later date, but it never seemed to materialize. Cheating was also a big thing; she cheated even when she wasn't exactly dieting, and when she was, she would lie in her own food journals. Kate, in reality, probably wasn't ready to lose weight, even if she was able.

And she wasn't really pushed to diet all that hard, unless you consider shame a motivator. Her mother was concerned for Kate's appearance and would make devastatingly hurtful comments such as, "You would be really beautiful if you would lose weight." She would also mention the diabetes that ran in the family. This all made Kate both angry and afraid. Her mother was saying, in not so subtle terms, you are ugly and bound to be sick. That anger and fear would turn to embarrassment and sadness when Kate would reflect on her current reality as a girl who didn't fit in, in so many ways.

It was long after that that Kate mentioned these episodes to her mother, particularly the facial expression of disgust. Her mother claims no memory, and insists it doesn't seem like something she would do. It's been more than twenty years that Kate has had that look her mother gave her etched into her memory; Kate remembers it clearly. That her mother denies it does not sit well. Nevertheless, their relationship has improved, but that is more a reflection of Kate being at greater peace with herself than a dramatic change in their dynamic. The more Kate takes care of herself, the more she is able to forgive her mother.

Kate had never exactly identified herself as having an eating disorder. Though she binged, she didn't purge. There were a few attempts, but nothing more. And she never transferred her bingeing on the snacks at home to her life outside of the house. She did not go in search of food out in the world when she was able. There are a few food items she stays away from now because they trigger the desire to overeat. Or, sometimes she will eat them anyway, because she genuinely wants to. She doesn't believe restricting food is productive.

In her mid-twenties Kate took up running again, and this time, although she was jiggling and wheezing and sweating and feeling very uncomfortable, she kept on going. She had learned to love using her body for how it makes her feel, rather than how it might transform her shape. As far as her shape goes, she is still large. She has at times been a bit slimmer and a bit bigger. She has also been smaller and less fit. She is in a good relationship, and because that takes priority, she will occasionally go home for a nice dinner and a cuddle rather than spend time in the gym. She focuses on balance.

Kate works with women in a community center and often encounters those who have been abused. She certainly relates to their struggle.

She has "come out" as a fat person, acknowledging it and allowing herself to enjoy her body, relationships, clothing, food, cooking, and simply living. "I spend a lot of time trying to think positively and productively about my body and my health and how it's connected to my wellness in general," Kate says. She is able to do this because she was diagnosed with post-traumatic stress disorder. If not, she wouldn't have had the opportunity to finally talk about all the things she was hiding from under her clothes—her disconnection, her anger and fear, her sadness and disappointment, her frustration, and even her size. Kate has found that perception is the key. It's not the size that matters.

PART FOUR

PART FOUR

18

UNINTENDED CONSEQUENCES STILL HURT

Stigmatization of Fat Children from a Sociological Perspective

BY PATTIE THOMAS, PHD

When I was a child—always the tomboy with the inevitable scraped knee or elbow—my dad would smile and say to me, "That can't hurt. I don't feel a thing." He was teasing, yet I admit when he said this, my first instinct, not understanding his intent, was to want to punch him. But once I had fussed a little and then laughed, I did feel better. It was clear that he cared. I realized, intuitively, his joke was an expression of empathy.

Social empathy is the ability to stand in another person's shoes and see the world from their point of view. We need empathy. From day one we struggle to communicate, which also means trying to figure out what our significant people are thinking— and in our early lives those people provide all our needs and nourishment—so clear expression is essential. In turn, caretakers of the young must exercise empathy, as sometimes our needs are not clear to us, and even when apparent they are often difficult to express in language. This doesn't end in childhood, either.

Social empathy in determining public policy, while equally important as it is in personal relationships, seems to be becoming more rare. Financial considerations, political maneuverings, and public persona too often shape policy, more than refection or even data. The goals of effective policy must first solve the intended problems, and second, not create new and perhaps worse problems. Thus, empathy is necessary in public policy making; it is a part of the data that will measure outcomes, and it is a part of assessing the probabilities of unintended consequences.

President Obama spoke a great deal about empathy, so much so that he has been taken to task by his opponents. He has often been accused of being "soft" because he employs empathy rather than reason. Both the president and Mrs. Obama have been quoted numerous times regarding bullying, and calling on policy-makers, and people in general, to help stop bullying.

This becomes ironic when you look at the first lady's flagship program "addressing childhood obesity:" the Let's Move! program. It has often reflected what people like to call "a war on fat." Such a war, particularly on children, will inevitably lead to bullying, and indeed has. Whether or not the intentions behind such policies are well meaning, what ultimately matters is the actual effects, which often do not match the intentions. Like any policy, if it creates more and even worse problems, it must be reevaluated and perhaps abandoned. That has not happened with Let's Move! or the war on childhood obesity.

It Starts with Stigmatization

Stigmatization is essentially the opposite of social empathy. Rather than seeing the world through another person's eyes, stigmatizing identifies someone as part of a group (a class, gender, race, ethnicity, size, religion, sexuality, and so forth), based upon a perception. It is irrelevant if the individual in question actually belongs to the group; it is the perception that counts. Then, based upon that perception, the stigmatized person is assumed to act in particular ways and have particular traits, usually based upon stereotypes of the group.

The person doing the stigmatizing does not truly observe or listen to the stigmatized individual and rather practices a kind of confirmation bias, where anything that matches the perception is regarded as "proof," and anything that deviates is either ignored or dismissed as "trying too hard" or "putting on airs." Sociologist Erving Goffman called this a *spoiled social identity*. While all of us try to manage the impressions others have of us, a stigmatized person cannot do anything to influence that impression. The person who stigmatizes refuses to see anything other than the social identity imposed upon the stigmatized person.

Three Fat Tales: Formula Stories of Childhood Obesity

Among the ways in which sociologists study social problems is an approach that seeks to outline and understand how a social problem is identified, ascribed meaning, and becomes a part of public discourse. One of the leading scholars in this approach is Donileen Loseke. In her book *Thinking About Social Problems*, Loseke points out that proponents of a particular view often create a story or narrative that helps audiences better understand the intended descriptions of problems and solutions. This framework essentially outlines the language of a particular social problem campaign. All campaigns use stories, so for instance framing the childhood obesity campaign a certain way does not necessarily suggest a problem with the campaign, but it does offer insights into ways of thinking that can then be assessed and analyzed.

In the winter of 2011–2012, Children's Healthcare of Atlanta conducted a controversial ad campaign called "Strong4Life," which featured pictures of larger children in what can best be described as a wanted-criminal-type pose. Included were slogans meant to be shocking, such as, "He has his father's eyes, his laugh, and maybe his diabetes." Or, "Chubby kids may not outlive their parents." A huge protest was launched against this campaign that spanned a political and cultural spectrum. Eventually, Children's Healthcare of Atlanta took the ads down, claiming they were going to do so anyway.

In the wake of the backlash, David L. Katz, MD, editor-in-chief of the journal *Childhood Obesity*, invited three professionals who work in the field of childhood obesity (Mary Murimi, professor of nutrition at Louisiana Tech University; Robert A. Pretlow, director of Weigh2Rock.com; and William Sears, associate clinical professor of pediatrics at UC Irvine) to discuss how best to bring "the issue of obesity, and in particular, childhood obesity, to the attention of the public to raise awareness of the problem and, presumably, provoke constructive responses." The transcript of this discussion was published in the April 2012 journal issue. The discussion provides useful insights into the thinking of the current efforts to "end childhood obesity," an effort many organizations often state as their purpose.

Loseke suggests that when this kind of rhetoric is used to describe a social problem, what she calls a *formula story* is developed. This *story* is called *formula* because there are consistent elements present, no matter what the topic of the discussion. Specifically, the story will have at least one of the following: a *victim*; a *villain*; a *condition*; and a *proposed solution*. These formula stories are useful in creating campaigns that convince audiences to support and act, but they can be limiting because they have a tendency to use exaggerated, even panicked, story lines and reduce complex aspects of life into simple ideas with generic solutions.

In the course of their discussion, Katz, Murimi, Pretlow, and Sears touch upon three formula stories that can be found often among childhood obesity researchers and activists.

1. Lifestyles

In this tale, the victim is a fat kid who is at the mercy of poor parenting. The villain or villains are either the parent or modern living that has led to a lifestyle of poor eating and exercise habits and a lack of knowledge of better choices. The conditions are based on two assumptions: First, fat kids obviously eat too much and exercise too little, and second, calorie restriction and better nutrition and exercise habits will lead to a smaller and therefore healthier body. The solution is to convince the parent that they must change the eating and exercise habits of their fat kids in order to make them normal size. Emphasis is placed on body size as a measure of success.

Illustrating this, Pretlow states in the discussion,

> I am a pediatrician, and I run an online weight-loss program for overweight kids. In attempting to avoid obesity and achieve healthy body weights in childhood, I think we need to focus on weight.... I applaud the Georgia ad campaign. We very much need to bring the issue of childhood overweight and obesity out into the open.

Additionally, Sears concludes,

> I am for anything that works. I think the positive side of the Strong4Life campaign in Georgia, where nearly 40 percent of children are overweight or obese, is its shock value. I also think that *Maggie Goes on a Diet* is an excellent book, because the moral is that Maggie, although obese, recognized it and took charge of her problem. She got lean, with "lean" meaning the right weight for one's body type, rather than underweight. For a child or a parent, reading that, it gives them hope.

Because the villain and victim are in such close relationship to each other and may both be in denial of the "real" problem, creating a shock to get their attention becomes an acceptable strategy. The assumption is that if parent and child were already aware of the problem they would have addressed it, and we would know this because the child would be at a "normal" weight.

2. Big Food

The victims, conditions, and solutions under the *big food* story are essentially the same as the *lifestyles* story. The difference is the villain. Processed foods that contain high-fructose corn syrup, the wrong kinds of fat, and "empty" calories, are vilified as the source of the rise in BMIs among children. This argument is two-pronged. First, the foods available are addictive. Second, fat kids are addicts.

To make this argument, most proponents, including Pretlow in the cited discussion, use a technique Loseke calls *piggybacking*. When a previous but somewhat unrelated campaign has been successful, new campaigns create parallel arguments. In the specific case, Pretlow outlines his "obesity as an addiction" approach, while acknowledging that research support for this parallel has not yet been developed, using the word "embryonic" to describe it. He nonetheless advocates it as a model that explains why diets do not work.

Sears supports Pretlow's assertion with a concept he calls *shaping young tastes*:

> Let's say you are giving advice to parents who are starting an infant on solid foods. What is happening at that stage in the average family? At six months of age, babies are given artificially sweetened, color- and flavor-enhanced food. That food tastes good, so these babies' "gut brains" become addicted to its taste and gut "feel." The brains in their heads get addicted to the serotonin release promoted by all that sweet stuff. So, we are beginning to addict babies to fattening foods at six months of age. If we could back up and get these babies addicted to the taste and gut feel of real food, such as with a "real food" campaign, we would have a good start.

Murimi completes the story and makes the connection to the villain by continuing the parallel story with addiction—specifically, smoking:

> Another important thing about the anti-smoking cam-
> paign was the change in policies of the environment....
> Changing the environment that affects the behavior is very
> important. That is the next step in childhood overweight
> and obesity campaigns. We need to talk to our food indus-
> tries about how they impact the environment through the
> foods they make available.

This formula story shifts the focus from blaming the people involved (caregiver/child) to blaming a villain about whom it is
much harder to argue. A successful social problems claim usually
involves a villain that lacks personality and sympathy. Blaming
parents, especially mothers, creates an immediate argument with
those who are leery of claims that parents must be perfect in order
to be good parents. Shifting the focus to an abstract entity avoids
such arguments. It is much less divisive to want to change the
for-profit food industry than the mother. Thus, the claim becomes
less controversial and easier to follow and accept.

In addition, the piggybacking-onto-addiction formula story continues a call for a change of behavior in the victims, even
without overtly blaming them. Addicts, after all, have come to be
regarded as "not to be blamed for their addiction," but once understanding that they have an "addictive personality," are expected to avoid those things that would trigger that addictive behavior.
Thus the diet and exercise aspects of the story remain intact.

3. Prevention

The main victim of the *prevention* formula story is the unborn
or neonatal child. Another victim is the normal-weight child who
might become overweight or obese if they or their parents are
not educated in correct choices. The villain is the mother or the
structural difficulties that the mother faces. The conditions and
solutions are similar to the other two formula stories, but the action that needs to be taken, the intervention, is said to be needed
much earlier in the parent-child experience.

Katz explains why he supports prevention strategies:

> As a preventive medicine specialist, I endorse [prevention, as described by Murimi] entirely. Although my own efforts in that particular area haven't had much traction, I have long believed in the importance of prenatal prevention of obesity, and I agree that one begins shaping the palate of a newborn with the maternal diet during pregnancy. So, I think we want the obstetricians as well as the pediatricians in on this to take advantage of that teachable moment during pregnancy.

This story has an added advantage over the others. One of the most important aspects of a successful victim in a formula story is that the victim is sympathetic, usually becoming a victim through no fault of his or her own. Prevention formula stories include normal-weight children as well as fat kids. The potential of becoming fatter even in the womb creates a victim who may fall prey to the condition but obviously, by virtue of not being born, has not, yet. No one can fault a fetus or neonatal child for the predicament. The prevention formula story also broadens the field for the social problems claim, giving the claims-maker moral authority—what is morally right and wrong—over any caregiver-child relationship, not limited to kids who are already fat.

While there is overlap in these three formula stories, they have the potential to lead to quite different public campaigns. The *lifestyles* story justifies shock campaigns meant to wake up families to impending dangers. The *big food* story suggests campaigns that address corporate decisions and possible regulation of ads and availability of some foods to kids. The *prevention* story leads to broad, sweeping campaigns aimed at all children and their caregivers, and allows for failures resulting from a lack of early intervention rather than just the diet and exercise solution.

In all three campaigns, however, the ultimate goal is to ensure that children are normal-sized, though there may be variations in the definitions of sizes, and the methods and the standards of success. In all three campaigns, a "troubled person" must be transformed into a "normal person." According to Loseke, when a social problem campaign emphasizes a troubled person, transformation to normal is always part of the story line. The troubled person is troubled due to what Loseke calls a *primary deviance*. Instead of fitting in and following the norms, the troubled person deviates from the norm in a specifically defined way. In this case, the troubled person is a fat child. This primary deviance is the focus of the solution of the campaign. Changing the troubled person, thus, requires a *secondary deviance*—a change of the troubled person into a normal person.

Unintended Consequences of Formula Stories

The problem with simplified, reductionist stories is that everyday life often does not work out as planned in the stories. Defining the primary deviance within the population of children is the first problem faced by these formula stories. One look at the ways in which "overweight" and "obese" categories have been developed for children show the difficulties in even discussing weight as a measurement of health. The definition of "overweight" and "obese" for adults are simple cutoff points in the BMI. But growing children make cutoffs difficult. To attempt to address this, percentiles based upon BMI and age are used. The 85th to 95th percentile of children are classified as overweight, and above the 95th percentile is obese.

The Centers for Disease Control, on their webpage *About BMI for Children and Teens* (at www.cdc.gov) explains why this has been deemed necessary:

> Although the BMI number is calculated the same way for children and adults, the criteria used to interpret the meaning of the BMI number for children and teens are different from those used for adults. For children and teens, BMI age- and sex-specific percentiles are used for two reasons: The amount of body fat changes with age. The amount of body fat differs between girls and boys.

The CDC BMI-for-age growth charts take into account these differences and allow translation of a BMI number into a percentile for a child's sex and age.... The interpretation of BMI-for-age varies by age and sex so if the children are not exactly the same age and of the same sex, the BMI numbers have different meanings. Calculating BMI-for-age for children of different ages and sexes may yield the same numeric result, but that number will fall at a different percentile for each child....

Fat kids are literally defined as those kids who have the top 15 percent BMI in their age cohort. Using percentiles guarantees there will always be overweight and obese kids, even if the actual number of children at these higher weights decreases. Percentiles are mathematical deviances. The primary deviance of "not-normal" is built into the discussion, and it is based not on health but on deviation from the average weight. The nature of human growth has made such standards necessary if percentiles are to be used, but that does not address the dilemma of arbitrariness.

Measuring the success of campaigns is also complicated by a difficulty in comparing "before and after." In order for a claim of success to be made, one must be able to show that the secondary deviance has been achieved (the child has become normal). Children grow up, sometimes at astonishing rates in the short term. So noting that a child is no longer in a certain percentile is a comparison to other children, but it does not necessarily demonstrate success of a solution. How are these children categorized as they grow older? Do a different set of children make up the higher percentile categories down the road? Percentiles do not inherently address these sorts of issues.

In addition, the complexities of individual weight set up an ultimate failure for these formula stories. People, including kids, are fat for a number of reasons. It is well established in the science that considering all fatness to be a matter of diet and exercise is problematic. The reasons for why we are fat or fatter remain under scientific scrutiny and debate, but what most scholars agree upon is that it not just a matter of calories-in/calories-out.

If kids are fat for a number of reasons, then diet and exercise explanations become too simple, and inaccurate. But if we need more complex explanations for the rise in weights of children, the social-problems claim of a troubled person who needs to be transformed into a normal person begins to lose moral authority.

For example, a growing body of scholarship suggests that changes in pollution and exposure to chemicals may explain over- all increases in weight. Bruce Bloomberg at UC Irvine has done work in this area, showing that rats exposed to organic chemicals widely used in plastics and pesticides were fatter, even when they ate far less than the rats not exposed.

Another non-energy-model explanation that's gaining some traction is in the field of epigenetics (very simply, the change in gene expressions caused by outside influences). A 2011 review of existing research by Herrara, Keildson, and Lindgren called "Genetics and Epigenetics of Obesity," published in *Maturitas*, concluded that while not enough research has been done yet to establish definite connections to environmental triggers of epigen- etic obesity susceptibility (something geneticists call "tags"), "it is likely that both genetic and environmental effects on epigenetics will in turn be associated with obesity."

These two explanations alone undermine the primary deviance of weight variation as a simple result of behavior, and the abil- ity to change the troubled person (fat kid) into the secondary deviance (normal weight kid). But there is still another layer of complexity that undermines the formula story of childhood obe- sity. The complexities of weight loss set up an ultimate fail for these formula stories. If poor diet and lack of exercise are not the culprit (no matter whether these habits resulted from poor educa- tion, addictive foods, or lack of early intervention), then working toward the secondary deviance through better diet and exercise habits will also ultimately fail.

Diets Do Not Work

Even within the discussion of anti-obesity campaigns, the child-hood obesity researchers themselves state this, more than once. Why diets do not work is debated, this ultimate reality is why the prevention formula story is preferred over the other two. After all, if early intervention means no diet necessary, then the pre-dicament of failure of dieting is avoided. But again, they still rely upon an underlying assumption that fatness comes exclusively from a lack in diet and exercise habits. How do we know that a kid doesn't have good habits? Because the kid is fat. How do we know that a kid has achieved good habits? Because the kid is smaller than she was.

The dismal failure of school interventions suggests how much on the wrong track these formula stories have been. A 2009 me-ta-study published in the *Canadian Medical Association Journal* examined eighteen school-based physical education intervention programs designed to reduce the weights of larger kids. The study concluded that their "meta-analysis has shown that school-based physical activity interventions do not improve body composi-tion." Though, the authors of this meta-analysis cite two studies that show promise of dietary intervention working. However, the studies they cite are short term, less than two-year studies. It is important to point out that while these exercise interventions did not result in changes in body composition, other health benefits were observed. Kids, no matter what their size or changes in size, were healthier when they exercised.

As Bacon and Aphramor pointed out in "Weight Science: Evaluating the Evidence for a Paradigm Shift," a meta-analysis of dietary interventions published in 2011 in *Nutrition Journal*, long-term dietary interventions are not successful in producing weight loss for most people, but often improvement in dietary habits do show an improvement in health:

> Health benefits associated with weight loss rarely show
> a dose response (in other words, people who lose small

amounts of weight generally get as much health benefit from the intervention as those who lose larger amounts). These data suggest that the behavior change as opposed to the weight loss itself may play a greater role in health improvement.... Long-term follow-up studies document that the majority of individuals regain virtually all of the weight that was lost during treatment, regardless of whether they maintain their diet or exercise program.

But these formula stories are ultimately about weight, not health. In these stories, the primary deviance and the path to the second-ary deviance is not in how a fat kid behaves but rather in how a fat kid looks. The use of BMI (ratio of height and weight) is always about how a person looks, not their behavior. BMI does not mea-sure anything about behavior. Deviance based upon looks moves us from health and well-being into the realm of stigmatization.

Bullying and Harassment as Unintended Consequences

In 2007, in *Psychological Bulletin*, Rebecca Puhl and Janet Ladner published "Stigma, Obesity and the Health of the Nation's Children," an extensive review of literature regarding bullying and harassment of overweight and obese youths, in which they connect anti-childhood-obesity initiatives to the unintended con-sequences of reinforcing weight stigma:

> Given the research presented in this review linking at-tributions about control and causality of body weight to negative stereotyping, and given the vulnerability of overweight and obese youths internalizing societal stigma and negative stereotypes, it is imperative to consider how messages should be framed to children about notions of personal responsibility for weight.

Puhl and Ladner, however, put the final nail in the anti-child-hood-obesity campaign's formula story. The worst unintended consequences of simplification in formula stories, according to Loseke, is a reproduction of the primary deviance instead of the creation of the secondary deviance.

Loseke uses the example of prison to illustrate how this works. Once a person has been convicted of a crime and sentenced to prison, they have been defined as having a primary deviance: The person is a criminal who should have been a law-abiding citizen. Prison is meant to be a deterrence that should lead to a secondary deviance: The criminal serves time and understands the consequences of his behavior. Upon leaving prison, the prisoner, consequently, should be motivated to be a law-abiding citizen. The problem lies in the nature of prisons. To punish, and therefore deter, prisons keep prisoners from the general population and put them in social contact only with other criminals. The result is often to create a more efficient and determined criminal, thus reinforcing the primary deviance rather than creating a secondary deviance. This is the ultimate failure.

Puhl and Ladner point out that reinforcing weight stigma has a profound consequence on the physical and mental health of the victims of weight stigma. In fact, some evidence exists that the negative health consequences of weight may be more related to the stigma of weight than the weight itself. "The health consequences common among obese children may partly result from the effects of discrimination."

The formula stories developed with the intent to address a supposed public-health issue—childhood obesity—not only may have simplified the conditions to the point that the measurement of success is based not on a child's health but upon how a child looks in comparison to other children his or her age; but the resulting solutions may also, in fact, have a detrimental effect on the health of the victims, thus ensuring that these children will suffer from the very health consequences that the formula stories claim to be trying to prevent. So not only will fat kids (primary deviance) not become thinner kids (secondary deviance) in the long run, but they also may indeed become sicker adults.

But Shouldn't We Do Something?

The first and foremost answer to this question may be a simple "No." Much of the rhetoric around the childhood-obesity epidemic is based upon tenuous assumptions about weight and health, and much of the data has been presented in percentages that exaggerate the actual changes that have occurred in the past thirty years.

In her book *Killer Fat*, Natale Boero demonstrates that the so-called obesity epidemic is a postmodern epidemic rather than a traditional one. Once reserved for communicable diseases, the word "epidemic" has come to have multiple meanings in public discourse and in public-health discourse. Boero's book outlines the financial and professional incentives that have taken over public-health initiatives, especially at the federal government level, in the past thirty years. The roots of the formula story of *lifestyle* can be seen in the politics of the Healthy People initiatives that began in the 1980s. By emphasizing diet and exercise over more expensive prevention programs such as health screenings, vaccinations, hygienic control, environmental improvements, and anti-poverty programs, Boero demonstrates that private interests are now able to sell more products, develop more extensive markets, and control research efforts in what seem to be ever-expanding ways.

One need only follow the money in the current Let's Move! campaign to see the market effects on the anti-childhood-obesity efforts. One of the major private supporters of Let's Move! is the Alliance for a Healthier Generation. According to their website, they have developed relationships (claiming not to accept funds from them) with a number of interesting "industry collaborations":

> We rely on our diverse partnerships to create the multi-faceted solutions we need to reverse the rates of childhood obesity. Though we welcome everyone to the table, we don't accept funds from entities with which we are negotiating solutions.

Engaging with companies in diverse industries can systemically improve access to healthier foods and beverages as well as physical activity for kids and their families. Through our efforts, leading food and beverage companies, group purchasing organizations, and technology companies have agreed to help America's schools serve healthier foods and beverages through agreements we've brokered.

These partnerships include a number of the names that play the part of villains in the *big food* formula story. Companies like Pepsico, Mars, Dr Pepper Snapple, Coca-Cola, ConAgra, Dole, and Tyson sit among the more expected health food, fitness, and health care companies. Why would companies that are often vilified in public discourse agree to join these efforts, even bragging about their participation in their marketing strategies? Because big food has always had a diet division. Diet products are big food products and anti-childhood-obesity efforts expand their diet products into marketing directly to more children.

Perhaps the most telling part of the Alliance for a Healthier Generation's website is what is not there. After a decade of successful alliances with schools and companies, if this approach were successfully turning fat kids (primary deviance) into thinner kids (secondary deviance), would they not be publishing that result somewhere? The closest miss is their "Wellness Stories" page and it merely outlines two of their school programs, with success being defined as the adoption of school lunches and exercise programs. There is no mention of weight loss or changes in body composition.

So, if they cannot demonstrate weight loss and they are emphasizing program changes, why mention weight at all? That is at the heart of the problem with the anti-childhood-obesity efforts. All kids benefit from the availability of healthier food choices and more exercise. Connecting these efforts to weight loss successfully achieves one thing only: the stigmatization of fat kids.

Take Two and Call Me in the Morning: Social Empathy

If anything needs to be done, it is promotion of more social empathy. The formula stories of the anti-childhood-obesity epidemic efforts focus on how children look as a measure of success, not their health. This is stigmatizing larger kids. The connection between stigmatization and health outcomes research suggests that weight stigma leads to many of the health problems associated with larger weights. Research on the increase of the hormone cytokines may even have identified the physiological reasons behind the stigma/health connection.

But even without the health connection, it doesn't take too much imagination to understand that being bullied, harassed, and stigmatized hurts. It hurts when it is happening and it hurts long after it happens. Puhl and Ladner suggest that these effects exist even if the child loses weight or grows into their weight. Once internalized, these hurtful messages outlive growth and childhood.

If we really care about the health of our children, then we need to promote social empathy and reduce social stigma.

Since social empathy seems to be innate, with babies either being born with or learning fairly early on how to see the world through the eyes of their significant others, some have suggested that rather than teach empathy, we may need to simply stop discouraging it in children. How to successfully encourage empathy is really too large a topic to address here. But one thing is certain, anti-childhood-obesity efforts encourage stigmatization. Whether intended or not, such efforts are hurting, not helping our kids, no matter what their size.

Dr. Pattie Thomas received her PhD in sociology of health and aging at University of Florida. She is currently a tenure-track sociology instructor at the College of Southern Nevada. Dr. Thomas is also presently an expert blogger at Psychology Today. Along with her collaborator, Carl Wilkerson, MBA, she has co-authored a sociological memoir, Taking Up Space, and is currently co-producing a documentary, User Friendly Vegas (SINdustry CITY Productions). More information on Dr. Thomas can be found at DrPattieThomas.com.

19

UNLIKELY SAVIOR

There is something about Sara that reminds one of a baby bird. Her voice is soft and gentle, and although modest in tenor, it expresses the import of her words. They are a plea for, and about, kindness. She sounds like the dander of a young bird feels. In listening, you can't help but want to touch her gently, with caution and compassion. You can't help but feel your heart swell, and love her.

Why no one noticed that when she was a child is impossible to imagine, and only makes the reality of it all the more devastating. That Sara wasn't nestled under a protective wing would make the staunchest cynic weep. And even for those of us who are just slightly hardened by life, her pain is practically unbearable. And that is only how the listener feels. Imagining how Sara must have felt is almost too much to bear.

Now, Sara works with children, and although she considers herself blessed, at first the idea terrified her. To be watched and judged by those who have the capacity to cut her to the quick, and who did torment her so mercilessly, seemed an insurmountable challenge. But now she is able to see them in their innocence—as sentient beings full of love, even for her, which she finds hard to believe, but is no less grateful for every day. She says her childhood was night, and sharing their childhood is day. When she interacts with children today, she is finally herself, a person she never was before.

Sara claims she has always been fat. Since the very day she was born. Upon reflection, she considers that, maybe, she was "normal" at age two or three, but even then all her eyes could see was fat. When she witnesses pictures of herself at four years old she is not sure whether she sees a fat child. Sara avoids pictures of herself, but her recollection is the preschooler might not have been quite so fat, but she isn't certain. However, by the time she was in her fifth year, there is no question about it: She was fat.

Fat means, in this case, larger than her classmates. Not as small. Perhaps a size or two bigger. But that was fat enough to make her feel fat and experience life as fat. And by second grade, she says, even objectively speaking, she was obese. She gained a size over her peers each year beginning in kindergarten, and by the time she was seven, even adults would have judged her as a problem, and they did.

Now, she says she knows that she is responsible for rising above the judgment, for taking care of herself and not expecting others to lead the way to acceptance. But as a child, she had no tools, she had no knowledge of self-determination, that self-esteem comes from within, that the outside may fight you until you are bloody and raw, figuratively, and sometimes literally, and that ultimately we must forge our own path. But what child knows this? Especially a child who was not raised to know, and perhaps not actually raised at all.

Sara grew up in a home with a sick mother. Her mother was sick in various ways, but her underlying illness was mental. She was, at the time of Sara's birth, undiagnosed with bipolar disorder; though *disorder* is a generic clinical term and does not exactly reflect the extent to which her behavior was dis-ordered. Her mother was profoundly troubled, and that trouble extended to her children. Sara has two brothers, the eldest of whom spent nine years alone being raised by her mother. She does not know what damage was done to him, or to be more clear, what abuse was dealt upon him, though she expects it was substantial, and by the time Sara came along, neither he nor her brother next in line had the capacity to protect her.

Her father was oblivious, in denial, or maybe just absent. He worked two jobs, from morning until evening and then from evening through night. He wasn't present to witness what was in fact, to be blunt, torture. He wasn't present physically, and he wasn't present emotionally. In retrospect she recognizes her father had a real hand in the devastation she lived, though at the time, by comparison, he was virtually a hero. It is easier to believe someone is a hero when they aren't present to demonstrate otherwise. And to be fair, he wasn't entirely running away from the scene of the crime; he also had to support it, financially. He had three children and a sick wife, and from a practical perspective, he may well have done the very best he could do simply struggling to keep them all alive. Sometimes our best isn't good enough, through no fault of our own.

As far as Sara's weight went, all her father did was remind her that she was fat and offer to buy her new clothes if she became un-fat. Her mother's tactics were more perverse, far more complex, and in truth not geared toward the notion of Sara becoming thinner. It was her mother's claim that she became fat when Sara was born, and not before. Before, she had a 20-inch waist; at least that was the fable. There is no way for Sara to know if that is true; there is no evidence. But that is the story Sara's mother told, which less than subtly expressed (not only because it was easy to intuit, but also because her mother would say it in no uncertain terms), Sara's mother considered Sara the reason she got fat. For better, and mostly worse, Sara's mother strongly identified with Sara as a fellow fat person, and her attempts to lose weight, or not to lose weight, were made to be a team effort. They were like a tandem bicycle—that's how Sara saw it—and she was a rider in the back who had no choice but to pedal.

There was, in essence, competitive eating and competitive dieting. Sara was a child and did as she was told, and when she was told that this week they would eat nothing but string beans, Sara too ate nothing but string beans. Or when at midnight on a Saturday, her mother determined it was time for a new fitness regime, Sara would be in front of the television in the living room exercising, as she was instructed. None of this made any sense to Sara, but these jags wouldn't last long. Mostly Sara and her mother neither dieted nor exercised and her mother remained fat, blamed Sara, and they both got fatter. To this day Sara has never been on a "real diet," but there is more about that to come.

So, for as long as she can remember, and even before she can remember, Sara was taught to hate her body, and it went more deeply than that. She was taught to hate herself for her mother's body, and for her mere existence on earth. The fact of the matter is there is far more to the story than blaming Sara for her mother's fat, or the odd moments of craze dieting. While a child can be devastated by that alone, Sara suffered far worse. Her mother, severely mentally ill, was also profoundly abusive. Emotionally, physically, and sexually.

It was noted that Sara was tortured, and that is an accurate portrayal. There are some things that are almost too difficult to talk about; Sara has only talked about them in therapy, and to tell this story. With respecting how deeply private her experiences were and still giving some hints for perspective—as a young child, a toddler and preschooler, Sara mother's found ways to cause Sara deep physical and emotional pain. This included sexual abuse, and not for prurient pleasure, but for sadistic satisfaction. What was done to Sara is as horrific as you can imagine. It involved doing things no child could understand, and nearly no adult could understand either. It was meant to cause pain, and as payback. It is a wonder Sara survived it intact, in any way, shape, or form. That she is as kind and lovable now as any kind and lovable person is a testament to her strength and character in ways words on a page don't quite express.

Sara's mother hated her. Sara's mother made that clear by stating it repeatedly, and by actions so unspeakable that they are almost never spoken about. Even forty years ago, in an age where parenting standards were quite different than today, if anyone had known, there would have been major consequences. So the fact that Sara hated her body, and herself altogether, is no surprise. It is difficult to imagine any other outcome that isn't devastatingly worse.

Thus started Sara's war with her body, and war on her body, though her body was but an innocent bystander, a scapegoat, and a poor substitution for who initiated that battle and deserved the defensive attack. Some opponents are too fierce to fight. It was a dragon against a baby bird. Sara lost many battles, but arguably, by surviving she won the war.

To add tragedy to devastation, at least as Sara remembers it, she was the only fat child among her peers. Children, and other adults, were not gentle with Sara and her body. Her teachers in school seemed to be disgusted by her, or that is how she perceived it. She was bullied mercilessly, but it probably wasn't just her body that made her a target. Adults bullied her too. The school nurse was scolding about diet and exercise, as were doctors and other authority figures. To her at that time, these authority figures were like gods, and these godlike beings made it crystal clear she was flawed; though they didn't offer any guidance. There were no tools given for the job she apparently was supposed to undertake. The only tool she knew, for any job, was food. The only thing she had access to was food. The only friend she trusted was food. The only weapon she bore was food. The only armor she had to protect her was food.

Though not all, not even most, fat children have a clear sense that food is for them armament, Sara is clear. But not all, or even most, children need armament as much as Sara did. That is clear to anyone.

Over the years Sara continued to get relatively larger. The pattern was the same: She would gain slightly during the school year and in the summers when at home with her mother; she would become 10, 20, or 30 pounds heavier. Part of it was having the time and unlimited access to the refrigerator, but underlying that was the lack of any other coping mechanism for being trapped in the abuse. In part she learned this way of self-soothing from her mother, who would do the same. Sara always had a house stocked full of what she considers junk food. Her father worked in the warehouse of a major commercial baker, and taking home boxes and bags was a perk of the job, a fact she was too humiliated to tell anyone she knew, because after all, it was evidence of her fat. Although Sara used food to both distract and comfort from a very early age, Sara wasn't concretely aware of this behavior (or that she was modeling her mother) until she was about thirteen or fourteen years old, when it all became extreme. Up until then, it was just her life.

When Sara was a young child her mother would often oversleep with depression, and there would be a mad rush to get the kids to school in the morning, which did not include a wholesome breakfast as seen on TV. Her brother, then in second grade, while Sara was in kindergarten, would make himself peanut butter and jelly crackers for the ride. She was too young to do the same for herself, and in the car her mother would force her brother to share—much to his displeasure. His anger terrified her, but the crackers comforted her, and also, she was hungry. Something as simple as receiving crackers from her brother caused her conflict. She was grateful, and afraid, and confused. To this day her brothers have difficulty disassociating Sara from her mother, as they both were fat, and that somehow made Sara guilty too. They have no relationship to speak of.

Though Sara got no weight "help" at home, in Sara's elementary school the "overweight" kids were singled out and put in a program with a nurse's oversight. They were weighed every week and made to keep food diaries. Sara was honest in hers, but she was too young to articulate it in a way to please the nurse. One special night the family priest came to her house for dinner; lasagna previously stored in the freezer was served. Sara didn't like it, it had freezer burn, and her mother let her have chicken instead. In her food diary she truthfully recorded that she had eaten both lasagna and chicken for dinner. This angered the school nurse. Two dishes for dinner?! But Sara was unable to explain; besides, no one cared for an explanation anyway. At seven, she learned a valuable lesson. She had to lie.

At somewhere around age twelve or thirteen, Sara took up overeating as an aggressive act—punishing herself. Her mother was again in the hospital and it was her birthday. During their visit, Sara's father presented a cake, which her mother refused to eat, because it was just one of those days. The cake was sent home with Sara while her father remained at the hospital. Alone with the cake, she made a determined decision to eat as much of that cake as she possibly could. One piece, then two, by the third it hurt so much she was physically incapable of ingesting more. Suddenly she became ashamed and frightened, and for the first time she tried to make herself vomit. She was unable. But what she realized she could do was eat so much that the pain from eating was all she felt, and nothing else. This was of surprisingly great comfort to her. The physical pain of being too full was a relief from any other pain she might be feeling. She now knew how to hurt her body with food in order to ease her mind. This was equal parts distraction and punishment, what she needed and felt she deserved. It was her first, but not her last, foray into self-harm.

She hated her family and she hated her schoolmates, who constantly picked on her for the size of her body and breasts. She progressively hated everyone more each year as she became fatter and more obviously female. But mostly, she hated herself. She tried other distractive self-punishment—drinking and smoking—but nothing was both soothing and punishing as food. Food was the friend and enemy she could count on and control. Sara believed that all the abuse she received, from the bullying to sexual abuse, was exactly what she deserved. It never occurred to her that she didn't deserve it. She was raised that way. You got what you deserved, and if what you got hurt you, you deserved to be hurt, and if it humiliated you, all the more deserved. And as in most cases of abuse, it was never to be discussed, because if it was, you knew what you deserved.

Not surprisingly, feeling inept at the rest of her life, Sara put everything she could into her schoolwork. She could learn to spell and write, and be a good student. It was the only thing she thought she could do. She couldn't play sports or make friends, or be loved. She didn't have the right clothes or haircut, or body. She felt inherently wrong. Born that way. But she could read and get a good grade. Though even that wasn't normal. Everyone else was normal, so she couldn't be.

Actually, not everyone was normal. She was aware her mother wasn't normal. Despite it being all she knew, Sara had an instinct that it wasn't normal to have to tiptoe through the house, or that her mother wouldn't get out of bed for weeks, or that she would never know if today was going to be the day her mother would be in a rage—and that it was anyone's guess which sibling would be punished for it. The entire family became super-listeners. They would note how her mother was walking; was she stomping about or did she seem to be drugged? Consequently, Sara learned to hide. And when she got old enough to have free access to it, she learned to hide with food.

By the time she was in high school, Sara had moved up to the attic and it was her regular practice to sneak down to the fridge and make herself something to smuggle upstairs. It was always something quick and easy that could be hidden in her clothes. A favorite was bologna sandwiches, which she would carry under her shirt. Or she would pull her sleeves over her hands and cover the contraband that way. She also favored whatever she could mix with hot water from her bathroom sink—jailhouse cooking. Ironically, there was no one monitoring her food, except her. Her parents weren't looking to stop her from eating more. Other than the odd week of string beans and cabbage soup years before, her mother wasn't dieting and wasn't expecting her to either. Her father wasn't present or aware. Sara was hiding her secret eating from herself. Or so it seems. And it wasn't the quantity that mattered so much as the act of subterfuge. She wasn't bingeing exactly, just eating, maybe a little bit more than someone else. But her perception of the entire situation was skewed by the reality of the entire situation.

It is very difficult to see the world clearly when the person you are supposed to be able to trust the most makes it crystal clear that, in her eyes, you are nothing.

Around this same time, Sara's mother was in therapy, and Sara unwittingly found an exercise from the psychiatrist. Her mother was to make a list of all the things she liked about her daughter. The few disjointed items made no sense; Sara could not recognize this person her mother supposedly liked. For instance, her mother claimed she liked that her daughter could knit. Sara could not knit. Sara hadn't the slightest idea who this person was that her mother thought her to be. Sara was a stranger to her own mother, who she already knew did not like her. And the feelings were mutual.

There were adults in Sara's life that she remembers fondly, though the bulk of time she spent with them was in her infancy. Her aunt and uncle were kind to her, and apparently took care of Sara when she was first born and her mother was unable. Sadly, Sara was an adult before she ever knew of this gesture. Had she known earlier, perhaps she could have reached out more herself. She has a few scattered memories, though, that help her to have some faith in humanity. One time while visiting, Sara asked for a snack and they gave her an apple. She was only about four and explained she couldn't eat it whole, and with the skin. Her uncle cheerfully cut the apple, and while he did he explained to her that the skin was the best part—the part with all the vitamins. This memory is clear in Sara's mind because it was the one time she recalls an adult lovingly explaining to her something about food. There was no judgment or condemnation, just a nice man teaching a little girl. Expressions of caring were few and far between for Sara.

Her feelings about her parents' seemingly total lack of concern for her weight is a source of conflict. Although she imagines being very resistant, there is a part of her that wishes they had introduced some sort of rational dieting, maybe took her to a doctor or therapist. She doesn't know exactly what she would have wanted, but she has a sense that if only they had nipped this in the bud when she was little, her life could have been very different. Sara doesn't actually believe diets are good for children, but she truly had no guidance, and with such a void, it is easy to understand why she fanaticizes that if only they had helped her lose the weight at the very beginning, perhaps her journey would not have been so grim. There was a time in college when she was very bitter about this lack of help. But in retrospect she knows that she would have gotten around any intervention. As she explains it, she clung to food like a life raft.

College was a bitter time for Sara. The process to get there was difficult. High school was an emotional obstacle course. Her peers were always cruel, and teenage boys seem to inherently know the art of social torture. There were hallways in school she would desperately avoid, and when she couldn't, she would walk head down, books to her chest, as quickly as possible. Down the gauntlet would ring, "Here comes the two-ton moose." She never dated. The girls were not so overt, but they showed their disgust through alienation and general contempt. In the sickest of teen ironies, Sara developed a reputation of being aloof and unfriendly. It's hard to say whether all of this was worse than middle school, where on the bus, boys would throw sticks at her, pummel her with dirt, and crumble cookies in her hair. It was so bad that even her parents felt the need to intervene. She got moved to a different bus. There they only taunted her with words, a whisper in the ear: "You are so fat!"

This was the precursor to college, so she was understandably full of trepidation. She wrangled out of her admissions interview, claiming she didn't have the funds for the trip. When her parents visited the campus the summer before school began, Sara declined to join. She was certain that if the people from the college saw her before it was too late, they would change their minds, rescind the scholarships—disallow her entry just on principle. For Sara this wasn't irrational teenage paranoia; it realistically reflects the attitudes she encountered her entire life.

Although college was not as aggressive a place as past schools, by this time she was just worn down. As she entered the first semester, she started cutting herself. She was self-injuring with razor blades. A fellow student caught Sara when her cutting just could no longer be hidden. She was reported. Sara was made to leave school in order to get help. Her parents arranged for her to see a colleague of her mother's psychiatrist. His first question: "Why are you doing this to your parents, why are you terrorizing them?" Despite this "help," she somehow managed to get the behavior under control and was allowed to return to school.

Sara refers to this as a funny story. It is many things, but not funny. Just prior to college Sara was contemplating her body and realized that the only part of herself that she found tolerable was the inside of her forearms and her wrists. This little section was all that she could accept of herself, with its pure pale skin and hint of blue veins showing through. It was the only beauty she recognized in all her form. This is where she took the razor blades, and cut. She aimed to destroy the only part of herself she could appreciate.

When asked how she managed to survive, Sara explains that she has acquired some tools. Through therapy and age, she has managed to become a relatively whole person. She remains large, though she has taught herself things about food and eating her parents did not. She works each day to become healthier in every way. She has never dieted. She doesn't believe she is able and doesn't care to test it. For much of her life, food is how she survived. These days she works not to be in love with what she eats, and not to see it as her best, and only, friend. But there is no denying that, in a very real way, food, and fat, saved her life—and she has an insightful respect for that.

For those who might believe that it did nothing but cause damage, that Sara is flawed because she believes food was her unlikely savior, they simply do not understand what it means to truly need to be saved.

20

NOW, GRAPEVINE!

Robert lived between two worlds, a thin one and a fat one, and in some regards, he still does. Robert was still a baby when his parents divorced, and despite having a baseball lineup of marriages between the two of them, there was a distinct quality in each of the homes when Robert was growing up. Each may have been tolerable independently, but traveling between them presented more than a small logistical difficulty. Somewhere along the road to the next visitation, Robert, it would seem, was supposed to either shed, or don, some skin.

Although there were various players on each team, two women were positioned as coach in Robert's life. Roberts's mother is of Mexican descent, and perhaps as Robert feels is stereotypically so, she had a tendency to serve and eat foods that might induce weight gain. Or, genetically, she comes from larger stock. Either way, food was plentiful at her house, delicious, and the people were round. Robert's stepmother for the majority of his youth, on the other hand, was, perhaps stereotypically so, tall, blond, and very thin, and she played a lot of tennis. She was, let's say, conservative in her meal preparation and eating habits, and displeased with too much roundness of form.

Until the eighth grade, Robert would travel back and forth between homes, preferring his mother's, where she was in essence a single mom, and life was full of joy. There were men living in the house at times, but the relationships were so short Robert

barely remembers their names. No matter, Robert and his mom
had a splendid time, if you like a fiesta—and Robert certainly did.
That's not to say it was ideal; Robert's mom worked a great deal
and there were times he was left to his own devices. But that was
not altogether bad either, particularly when compared to the regime his stepmother instituted. With Robert's stepmother, things
were a bit more "buttoned up." Chores, and exercise, and eating,
were all part of a master plan, or at least there was a master behind the planning.

Robert says he has never really been thin. He has a big frame.
Though not tall, as an adult, a bit over five feet eight inches, he's
broad-shouldered, wide-chested, solid. He had a growth spurt at
one point and was the tallest of his friends, but that leveled off
and left him low to the ground and solid. Just like, not terribly
surprisingly, his mom. Robert's stepmother might have preferred
he had her genetics—but that would have required a relationship
of the genes.

At around the age of seven or eight, Robert started to put on
some weight. By nine years old, he says he was a pretty thick
kid. He didn't realize how much so until he changed schools and
his new peers mocked him for wearing pads while playing flag
football, when he wasn't. It was also then that the dichotomy of
the two households became more tense, or Robert became more
cognizant of it. His awareness wasn't entirely coincidental; it was
at that point his stepmother initiated her weight-loss and exercise
regime—which was serious business, albeit with major flaws to
the business plan.

Elementary and middle school seems to be a difficult time for
larger kids, particularly boys in sports. Their saving grace: football.
But that doesn't come until high school, when the bigger they are,
the harder others fall. Before boys are free to pummel each other
with impunity, there is not all that much for a bigger boy to do.
At Robert's new school, which he started in the fourth grade, all
the other boys seemed to be in really good shape. Every single one
of them was athletic, or at least it appeared that way to Robert. If

there were any husky or nerdy kids, they were assimilated into the mix of boys who had for the most part known each other since kindergarten. Robert was an outlier, and the fact that he was slow, got tired easily, was uncoordinated, or at the very least, fat, did not make life easier. He found his stride in high school football and then rugby, but that's another story. Needless to say, he was teased.

That was when his well-intentioned stepmother became a sort of ad-hoc coach, though whatever she was coaching him for, Robert would not have played that sport in public. In everyday life, there is not much call for a nine-year-old boy to be the star in a competitive game of *Sweatin' to the Oldies*, as much as Richard Simmons might enjoy that. Robert describes his stepmother as "cruel but not evil." That seems to mean she was tough on him, but her intentions were good. Though the discomfort at his father's house wasn't entirely his stepmother's doing. Robert was expected to "keep his back a little straighter" with his dad. "Moms are sweet and loving, but you try to act a little better in front of your dad; I tried to keep myself in line." However strict with his son, his dad was kind of a pushover when it came to the women in his life, and if his wife told his son to jump, Robert's father said "How high?"

Robert's stepmother had a two-pronged plan. It was pretty standard stuff: Diet and exercise. There were just some small peculiarities that made the endeavor a little more humiliating than necessary. Whether that was intentional or not is hard to know. First of all, there was the water. Robert was required to drink a specific amount of water each day, a very specific amount, and thanks to his portable Teenage Mutant Ninja Turtle water bottle at the ready, there were no excuses for dehydration. Robert was required to carry that bottle everywhere. That meant at school, when hanging out with friends, on trips, and vacations. Obviously, Robert's friends found this ridiculous and were not shy in saying so. Who can blame them? During that trip to Sea World, Robert is fairly certain the dolphins were mocking him, and they probably were.

On the other hand, Robert's stepmother believed in moderation when it came to eating. There were plenty of fruits and vegetables, and there is nothing wrong with that. But whatever the meal, Robert was in some kind of training, with the aim of desiring to eat less. He had to leave a bite on his plate, and then two. He was given a goal: Leave a cup of food uneaten. That's what he remembers, and he remembers it seemed like a lot. It's not that he was served too much, or that he was to stop eating when he quenched his hunger. It was merely an exercise in preventing perceived gluttony. Certainly Robert's stepmother didn't invent this dieting technique, but it was confusing to a little boy to be forced to stop eating before the end of the meal, just as it was for those being reminded of the starving children in a foreign land to justify a clean plate. Food wasn't to satiate, it was a morality lesson—and while morality should be taught, these methods were mostly effective in generating guilt, and disordered eating.

Unquestionably, the meals were stressful. Robert would be constantly reminded to slow down, which was difficult because he was ravenously hungry. He would sit with his head hanging, waiting for the next bite to fill his empty stomach. Leaving a bit wasn't an easy feat because in reality, he wasn't forgoing excess, he was dieting, and dieting means eating less than the body signals the need to eat. Robert didn't leave the table full, and really, he was hungry a lot of the time. Eventually he did crave less, he thinks, but he's not entirely sure. Signals may have become crossed.

Then, when it came to treats, the only allowable variety were dietetic. Snackwells, the Nabisco food-product for the weight conscious, and fat-free Jell-O were the "fun foods." Pure indulgence. Basically, Robert was being taught to eat like a middle-aged woman in the pages of *Redbook* or *Good Housekeeping*. Whether there is anything inherently wrong with that is a matter of perception, one supposes. But it's still a peculiar way to raise a preadolescent boy, and don't think Robert didn't know that.

But the worst, the undeniably worst, were the daily workouts. Robert was encouraged to play sports, and he did. He was signed up for soccer, though he had no particular interest in the game. There was a lot of running involved so it was deemed a good cardio workout, which is all well and good, except that when it is presented as such to a ten-year-old boy, it does not make the endeavor eminently appealing. Nonetheless, if that were it, okay. But it wasn't. Robert also had a schedule, which his stepmother shared, of exercise tapes and workout dance videos. Morning routines were half an hour and evening workouts went on for forty-five to sixty minutes. The rotation included VHS *Mousercise* exercise tapes for kids, compliments of Disney, and the more adult Richard Simmons library including such favorites as *Disco Sweat* and *Supersweatin': Party Off the Pounds*. Sadly, Robert is no longer a fan of the O'Jays.

To say this was embarrassing does not do the experience justice. The whole thing was presented as a regular chore, included on Robert's chore sheet, along with taking out the garbage and drying the dinner dishes. Stars and ultimately rewards were given for successful completion. Although Robert couldn't be certain every boy in the neighborhood wasn't also Grapevining with their mother figures, it seemed highly unlikely, even to a kid. He certainly didn't dare to ask his buddies for confirmation.

Robert's father did not join in on the aerobicize or the idiosyncratic dieting practices. He, too, was a big guy; Robert inherited that genetic predisposition from both sides of the family. Robert's father's weight did fluctuate, so he apparently did engage in some type of regime, but it was not all that apparent to Robert. His father had a stationary bike and was a competent racquetball player, so Robert had heard. He also had a small gym in the garage, though there were no father-son workouts. Beyond that, his father kept to himself on these matters, which was not altogether comfortable for Robert because Robert was in a humiliating situation, and he knew his father knew, and knew his father knew he knew. Robert describes the dynamic as having a "mental strain," which would continue to impact him throughout his life. He also claims there were health rewards, so in retrospect it was conflicting. Robert did see himself as a fat kid, which was detrimental, so these tactics, however uncomfortable, were effective, at least in some regards.

Although Robert certainly didn't publicize his daily jazzercise, the other kids very likely knew he was on some kind of a diet. All they had to do was look at his lunch. First of all, he nearly always brought his own, and it's difficult to hide a TMNT water bottle no matter how hard you try. Also, most of the other kids got to buy their lunch, at least some of the time. The school offered standard lunchroom fare: hamburgers, hot dogs, pizza, and also fruit, cookies with oatmeal, and milk for good measure. Some of his friends bought their lunch every day, and while that is not necessarily something to be proud of, when you're a kid in the lunchroom, you're proud of it. Maybe once a month, Robert would get the opportunity to buy his lunch—a big deal in the competitive world of random things that make you feel as cool as everyone else. To do this, Robert would frequently use his own money to buy the school lunch and throw out his bag of nutritious rations. Pizza day! Needless to say, he didn't tell his stepmother.

This sort of mentality bled into life when he went to live with his mother, only to a much greater extreme. There were no food restrictions at his mom's, which would have been fine, except that he would arrive there feeling resentful and deprived, not to mention hungry. When at his mother's he would gorge, knowing full well he wasn't going to eat that well the next week. He had to make up for lost time. So from week to week, Robert would be living in a surreal *Woman's Day* boot camp and then have access to all the burritos he could stomach. Not only was that physically unhealthy and an eating disorder in the making, but it also inspired quite a bit of frustration and guilt. Every week at his father's felt like starting over, as if he had failed and was back to square one. But that didn't help a kid maintain moderation when there was a food free-for-all in the off weeks.

Additionally, Robert found ways to circumvent his stepmother's protocol, even at her house. Getting his pudgy hands on some forbidden candy, he would eat it in the bathroom and flush the wrapper down the toilet. And when Halloween came around, Robert would wake up in the middle of the night to sneak candy, then go back to sleep. That was a caper because the candy was monitored, so Robert would scheme: Take the candy out of the bag surreptitiously, hide it somewhere, and then throw the wrapper evidence out the window. It's not like he got away with it, either. There was at least one incident with a plumber, clogged pipes, and accusations of illegal flushing. Not to mention someone had to clean up the yard.

Robert attempted to talk with his father about the untenable stepmother situation, but dad seemed to have blinders on, or just didn't want to deal with it, or perhaps approved of her methods—not for himself, mind you, but for his son. Eventually, Robert's dad got an inkling that things were a little extreme and there were some closed-door discussions. His stepmother let up, but just a bit. His father was well aware that Robert was embarrassed and frustrated, but it is unclear if the discussions were a result of empathy for the boy, concern, or just being tired of hearing about it. Of course Robert's father wanted the best for his son, but wanting and acting on that desire are not necessarily the same thing. Besides, Robert's father was a fat guy too, so what did he know about raising a healthy child?

It's difficult to say what was the worst part of the situation, considering it was full of parts that could easily have been the worst. But what happens in public always seems to hang on, for a long, long time. It was during those incidents when Robert's stepmother's good intentions came into question—and there is no better time to question good intentions than the holidays. Robert's family, particularly his stepfamily, was full of young athletes. Some even got drafted onto professional teams. Making assumptions about motivation after the fact can be dicey, but it's probably fair to say Robert's stepmother, with no children of her own—would-be tall, blond, very thin, and playing lots of tennis children—may have been a bit jealous of her relations. But whatever the reasons, her control on Robert was heightened at these gatherings.

During one Christmas in particular, the family had a buffet and Robert was keen on having the good stuff, except his parents were shoveling all this healthy food on his plate, and Robert wanted no part of it. He was just a boy, and the other boys got to eat what they wanted. He threw enough of a fit that his father escorted him out of the room. Returning, his dad lied about Robert's emotions, blaming them on the recent passing of his grandmother. Calmed, Robert went through the line himself and filled his plate with Christmas goodies. To add insult to insult, when he got back to the dining table, his father and stepmother, tag teaming, sent him right back where he came from, to exchange the eats. It was a spectacle. Robert was mortified. And pissed. Though in talking about it, less pissed than a lot of people would be. He acknowledges his own part in the debacle, begging the question: Is a little kid supposed to have the kind of discipline and self-control that was expected of him? For that matter, shouldn't an adult have the kind of discipline and self-control required to avoid instigating a child?

Eventually, Robert both grew into his weight and became more of an athlete. He played sports more seriously in high school and by college was quite competitive, though he was born with his body type and that hasn't changed. And his concern about his weight hasn't changed. In fact, in some regards it's worse, because now, all of the anxieties and pressures are his own.

It would probably be going too far to say Robert has a clinical "disorder," though that would be for a clinician to determine, but as difficult as it is for women to fully disclose their food and body issues, it is even more so for men.

No one in his life condemns him for his size anymore; no one monitors what he eats, or how much exercise he gets. No one, that is, except himself. Regardless, Robert remains self-conscious. He becomes particularly sensitive about his body if he's been out, had a few beers, maybe some pub food. Then he looks in the mirror and sees a fat man, a man that is out of shape. Thoughts run through his mind: "I'm such a fat ass, I need to lose 10 pounds." He isn't, and he doesn't. In fact his weight has been rock steady for many years. But when he has these thoughts they are powerful, and emasculating. "I sound like such a woman." Which would probably be all right if the womanly thoughts weren't inherently destructive.

When Robert gets into this state of mind, or if he is displeased with himself for whatever reason, he reacts by punishing himself the same way he felt punished as a child. After all, that is how he was trained. He doesn't binge eat—that was rebellion. He binge exercises, because that was his punishment for bad behavior. Robert runs regularly to stay fit, but at these times of insecurity he runs to run. He will run eight miles and not realize he has done so. Recently, he ran ten miles and wasn't aware of the distance until he returned home. The longest he had ever run prior to that was a half marathon, but in a half-marathon setting. This run was unsupported and unaware, and to him in retrospect, unfathomable.

Mystified, Robert has given this a great deal of thought. He realizes that he punishes himself with exercise. He pushes himself until it hurts. He recalls going back to his father's house after a week of freedom with his mom, and the anticipation of the coming punishment. He knew he was out of control while with his mother, and now comes the discipline, which he despised, but thought perhaps he deserved.

This rationale extends beyond the deeds he does to himself. He takes measures when his bad behavior affects only himself, but the measures are even more severe if he has been bad toward someone else. He is married now and there is distance in the relationship. He knows he is disconnected and rather than address the problems in the dynamic, he runs. Sometimes instead, he goes to the gym and lifts for two hours, but symbolically, he is running. Sometimes he goes to the gym and works out so hard his wife has to pick him up because he is unable to manage on his own. He has run until he literally can't run anymore. He runs until he is figuratively, and even literally, paralyzed.

His wife knows little about what he went through as a child. He has mentioned it in jest, but is hesitant to tell the whole story.

He fears it will hurt her. He doesn't mention whether it will hurt him. He has a Richard Simmons phobia, literally. Just the name sends shivers, and ironically, he had the displeasure of seeing Simmons once at an event. Robert fled. His wife knows that. She knows he was a heavy kid and lost weight. She knows there is some resentment. But she doesn't know the extent of the impact.

Robert is sensitive about his wife's weight. She is an athlete, a marathon runner, and a former Marine. She also eats, as Robert perceives it, nonstop. Far more than he does. Though she has virtually no body fat, her eating makes Robert angry. Sometimes he complains about the money it costs to feed her, but that is not the true issue. He's just jealous. He resents her. And, he's afraid she might get fat. Not a rational fear with this woman at this point, but if she did, it would cause devastation. It has happened before. In a previous relationship, a woman put on weight. She did not mind, but he was very troubled. It wasn't even a lack of attraction that caused the real rift, it was what putting on weight symbolized for Robert. It represents being out of control, of not having control, of needing to be controlled by others. And that is unacceptable.

Robert doesn't dislike fat people, but he feels sorry for them. He feels both a sympathy and an empathy. And he admits, he feels judgmental. He thinks about all the work he does to keep the weight off and he wonders why they don't aspire to the same goals. "How could you let yourself get to that point?" And with fat kids: "They never had a chance." He notices large children like he has a homing device. He will see them in a crowd, down the street, across the park. He sees every kid that reminds him of himself, and then the parents, and they anger him.

He understands about fat stigma, he understands about genetics. That's all clouded by experience, and perhaps a touch of Stockholm syndrome. He hopes that if he has children, they have his wife's genes. If not, he won't be as strict with them, he will be more encouraging and participatory. He knows that his attempts at rebellion probably increased his weight. He doesn't want that.

He doesn't want to perpetuate a vicious cycle. Frankly, it scares him to think about it. He doesn't actually know what he would do. He knows he won't make them dance to the oldies, but what about a dance to a different tune? Whatever the songs, he's still dancing.

21

FAT PANTS FOREVER

Meg feels as though she has been overweight so long, she must have been fat in the womb. She isn't sure exactly when she first became conscious of it, but by the time she was in kindergarten, she knew she was larger than normal. She is certain of that. By the fifth grade, Meg had a tangible measurement of comparison. She wore a size 16, and there is no doubt hers were the largest pants in the class. Certainly by then the kids were saying mean things to her about her size, and she felt bad every time they did. But if that was their goal, it really wasn't necessary for them to make fun of her. She felt bad about how she looked, regardless of what they said. Meg desperately wanted to be thinner. So much so that she put herself on a diet and managed to lose a lot of weight before going into the sixth grade. She wasn't compelled to lose weight by anyone else—though her doctor did suggest she eat things like fruit instead of crackers, and her mother offered to pay for Jenny Craig—but Meg initiated it on her own. She created what she thought was a healthy meal and exercise plan, and she dieted.

For whatever reason, Meg wasn't interested in Jenny Craig. She was headstrong and determined she knew what was best for her soon-to-be sixth-grade body. She ate less, though with no particular focus on nutrition, and worked out with the judicious guidance of television exercise videos. Meg lost weight, and she sustained that weight loss for a significant amount of time, considering. But, as inevitability would have it, as she approached high school, she began to put the weight back on. She was growing as well, of course, so the weight gain was in part a consequence of that, but at the time, Meg wasn't in the head-space to distinguish growth weight and fat weight. Numbers on the scale were numbers on the scale, and they said all Meg needed to know. So it was in high school that Meg began to use more creative methods for weight loss. Her go-to course for the removal of excess was laxatives, in copious amounts. Bulimia via the bowels lasted for several years.

Meg took her weight very personally, in that she believed it was personally her own damn fault. Whatever weight Meg happened to be at the time as a child or a teen, if she was picked on for it, she felt that's what she deserved. To her, the teasing wasn't bullying, as we often call it now. Bullying happens to those who don't deserve it. Bullying is also more intense and targeted, perhaps violent, or at least aggressive. Meg was merely teased. Someone might make a derogatory comment, and then laugh. It's not that it wasn't painful. It was tremendously painful, but not so much because Meg was the butt of a joke, but rather, whatever they said about her size, she tended to agree. The teasing was merely redundant. What they were thinking about her, she thought worse. What they said, the voices in her head had been saying longer and more assertively. She knew others found her homely—it didn't need to be said. The fact is, it was said in every aspect of society that spoke of and to girls, and how they are supposed to appear. This may have influenced her self-perceptions just a bit. But regardless, she agreed.

Perhaps it is an overstatement to say she felt she deserved it. More likely, she believed it was just an expression of truth. "Of course people are going to make fun of me because I'm larger. It wasn't okay or right, but it was expected." No one had a more negative attitude toward Meg's being fat than Meg. She remembers this sense of herself, and how repercussions were to be expected, as early as kindergarten. It isn't an actual memory of events; it's a memory of her mother telling her the events occurred. Why her mother told her this, she cannot remember. It's unsettling that the messages were relayed by her mother, but it wasn't something she didn't already know. Instinct.

What Meg does remember firsthand is her weight in the second grade. She was 120 pounds. The average "normal" weight for a seven-year-old girl is about half that. She may not have known the particulars, but she certainly knew she wasn't "normal." They weighed the children in school, for gym class, and made certain the kids knew their results. Meg held on to that number so tightly it practically made her bleed. One hundred and twenty. It became the representative number for all things big. The teacher asked her class to guess the weight of the biggest pumpkin, an enormous, huge, mammoth pumpkin. One hundred and twenty pounds. Meg was the same weight as the pumpkin. "I was as large as the largest pumpkin.... I felt bad, I wished I wasn't that large. I was larger than the people around me—I was larger than some adults. I was always aware of that. Even when I was doing other things, I never lost track of being 120 pounds." As large as the largest pumpkin.

Meg still never forgets, though she is no longer fat. She may well weigh 120 pounds, but now, that's not fat. It doesn't matter. She feels fat. She frequently thinks about being smaller than she is. Every time she puts on a pair of jeans, as she pulls them up, she wonders if she's as big as a pumpkin. Even when she is smaller, she feels bigger. That light came on when she was so young, it never turns off. It may dim, when her size diminishes, but it never turns off. And to be clear about the light, it's not because she was fat so young, it's because she felt bad about being fat so young. The light does not illuminate fatness, it illuminates shame.

Meg believes that her weight as a child was at least in part genetic. Both of her parents are overweight. "They don't partic-ularly look for healthy food, though, so I think both things were involved." Meg asked her mother why she was fed those foods, when the result made her feel so terrible. "That's all you liked; you wouldn't eat vegetables or healthier foods." Meg blames herself for that—she should have known better. Upon greater reflection, however, Meg isn't certain how large her parents were. There were periods when her mom was larger, but Meg as a child outsized her mother's childhood size. Meg isn't sure whether she actually ate a great deal of junk food, particularly compared to other children. Compared to what she eats now, there were more crackers and chips, less fruit, more meat. She has no idea if she ate more than the other children. There really is no way to know.

She brought her lunch to school most days, but once a week was hot-lunch day. She recalls buying two cheeseburgers when the other children would buy one. She remembers that, and trying to hide the second burger, so no one would know. Her mother knew. The meals were prepaid and her mother paid for two—after Meg asked for them. She thinks she remembers asking because she was hungry. But she's not entirely sure. She does know it was the first or second grade.

Meg, in retrospect, and upon current reflection, doesn't think she always eats because she is objectively hungry. But she isn't certain of that either. "It seems like a weird thing not to know." Most likely, Meg doesn't always eat because she is objectively hungry—but that is based on the fact that for most people, not every morsel consumed is in response to hunger. Somehow, when Meg makes this blind choice—often the same choice made by others—it's worse.

Other than not wanting her schoolmates to know she ate a second cheeseburger, Meg was not a closet eater. She never hid the food she ate. She did binge, but she did so out in the open, right in front of her mother. In middle school, for instance, after she had lost all that weight on her self-made diet, Meg would think, "I lost all this weight, now I want to eat." She would take a box of cookies, or whatever else was around that was good cheat food, and consume it all. It was not surreptitious, and her mother didn't say a word. Her mother didn't tell her it was unhealthy, or would cause her to gain weight, or ask her if something was emotionally awry. Not even an "is there something you want to talk about, Meg?" Meg seems to resent this; at least that is how it appears when she discusses it. At the very least, she finds it curious, and perhaps a sign of less-than-stellar parenting. But if her mother had intervened, she might have resented that, too.

Meg's parents weren't aware of everything she did. They didn't know about her extreme dieting attempts or laxative use. Though she suspects they knew more than they let on. Here's the conundrum: In all likelihood, Meg would have been displeased either way. Just based on what tends to happen, when parents intervene in the child's weight-loss protocol, the child feels controlled. When they don't, the child feels abandoned. And either way, body-image issues and eating disorders frequently follow. It's a tough call for everyone, and there doesn't seem to be one entirely right answer, at least not an easy one, or one that works across the board.

Nonetheless, Meg feels her parents witnessed, and were a party to, some pretty unhealthy stuff—eating too much fatty food, not eating enough fruits and vegetables, awareness of the binge eating—not to mention whatever they knew about Meg, that Meg didn't know they knew. "And they didn't express concern or even mention anything, so yeah, I do think if my mom knew how bad it felt to be larger—and whenever I was upset about it, she said she did, that she experienced it too so she understood—I do wish she had done something to help me, either to not feel that way and be more confident, or lose weight. I don't feel she did that. So yeah, I would say that I am still a bit angry." It is not all that surprising that their relationship isn't particularly good now.

Even though Meg doesn't feel her parents were as emotionally available or supportive as she would have liked, she doesn't make a direct connection to that and food. She wasn't an emotional eater as a response to her relationship with her parents. But they didn't offer her guidance, and she wanted that. They ate whatever they wanted without concern for weight. From Meg's perspective, her parents didn't care about their own size, or hers. Which is probably true, and may or may not be a bad thing. But since Meg felt differently, she was on her own. She felt she was on her own emotionally, in general. Her parents expressed that Meg was too sensitive, that she was over-emotional, and overreacting. They behaved as if they didn't know that children teased her, or that she disliked being large. Meg thinks they knew, though it's hard to say to what extent they knew, because they weren't paying very close attention.

It's not like her parents tried to prevent Meg from losing weight, and they didn't attempt to sabotage her. They were merely disconnected. When Meg began her pre-sixth-grade diet strategy, they let her exercise in front of the television in the living room and never forced her to eat food she didn't want. But there was an inertia. As Meg dieted, she would get very hungry for dinner and would, from her mother's view, pester her about when the meal was to come. So Meg's diet was at times a mild irritation, but there was no great drama. She says they were "passively accommodating."

Later on, Meg's mother would begin to employ more aggressive tactics, which seemed, at least on some level, bent on sabotaging her daughter. Though that probably wasn't her intention, directly. Meg's mother would do things like send her giant boxes of chocolate on Valentine's Day—which seems thoughtful, except Meg didn't want them, and she told her mother so. But her mother appears unable to find another way to express her love, or she doesn't want to try. So Meg continues to receive chocolate she has asked not to be sent. She wonders if her mother forgets about Meg's objection, but that would mean it's not important enough to her to remember, which is a pretty unsatisfying alternative.

It was in the seventh grade that Meg began coming home from school to eat an entire box of cookies. In middle school, she lost the weight, sixth grade she managed to maintain it, and by seventh grade, the all-so-common response to restricting food occurred: reactive eating. The resulting weight gain was totally unacceptable to Meg, but the pattern had begun, and once it starts, it's very difficult to stop. Meg resorted to what many binge eaters resort to—purging the excess food. In her case, she used laxatives. That started when she was sixteen, in her third year of high school. She learned about laxative use for expelling binge-eaten foods from, of all places, a textbook from health class. There was a story about some young woman who used laxatives to control her weight. Of course, the moral was that doing so was an awful idea and terribly unhealthy. It also served as a how-to manual in the process.

Meg's reaction to the story: What a great idea! Now I can eat what I want and not gain weight. Her laxative use, or abuse, lasted through the remainder of high school and into community college. As with many medications, the body builds up a tolerance, so more and more is required to do the same job. Meg continued to increase her dose—reaching a full family-size package of thirty at a time, which is not uncommon—she bought her supply from multiple stores so as to not to arouse suspicion, which is also not uncommon. Unsurprisingly, it became increasingly difficult for Meg to function. She weaned off laxatives, mostly out of necessity. Meg would have to get up in the morning and leave the house, go to school or work. That's difficult to do tied to the toilet. It wasn't so much a concerted effort to stop as much as practical reality got in the way. She received no therapy or treatment.

No one knew about this behavior, or if they did, they didn't say so. She shared a bathroom with her brother, but he either didn't know, or didn't want to know. It was all a secret. She likes to believe that her parents never found out, because if they had, they didn't express any concern whatsoever, and that seems worse than them not knowing.

A little later, Meg spent some time living in Eastern Europe. Their attitude toward women's bodies seemed to Meg to be very different. Although they were generally smaller than Americans, and at least appeared healthier, there was not so much of a stigma attached to weight. Appearance, and thinness, were less important. Even the actors and otherwise famous people looked more like everyone else. That is Meg's impression, but regardless of whether it was true across the board, she felt judged much less. One time shopping for pants in a market, an old woman pointed to Meg's item and said to a friend, "She's looking at those pants for fat girls." At first Meg was taken aback at her boldness, and rudeness, but then she realized the woman was just pointing out a fact. She wasn't saying that a "bad" girl needs fat pants—merely that they were made for a fat girl. Her intention was no different than if she were noting pants for a baby, or a child, or a man, or any other human being who might need such an item. Nothing more, nothing less. That was difficult for Meg to process, because whenever she thought of buying clothes for a fat girl, the next thing on her mind was how much she wanted to be thinner.

Meg's time in Eastern Europe was the only period in which she really dated. She had a boyfriend while there. But hadn't in high school, or since her return from abroad. "I don't think most American guys found me attractive then, or do now, and I think the fact that there is less focus on weight in Eastern Europe is why." Meg acknowledges that some of that may be perception rather than reality. "It might be related to confidence, and I don't feel confident, so I don't seem open to men who are attracted to me. But I'm thirty-three and still single; some of it's perception, but it must also be my size."

Here's the rub—Meg isn't fat, not by most anyone's standards but her own. She wears a size 6. In fifth grade she wore a size 16. At thirty-three she wears a 6. At five feet five inches tall, she wears a size 6. She's also an athlete, which of course doesn't mean she's not fat, but she's not fat. "It feels like I'm fat. I am a lot more focused on it now. I feel very large. I feel like I eat a lot and I feel like I'm gaining weight. I am worried about it more so now than I did when I was larger. Maybe that sounds funny; I'm not that large now and objectively I know that, but it's in the forefront of my mind still."

Actually, that doesn't sound funny at all. It sounds like body dysmorphia, or at least having a warped perspective on her actual appearance. And there is nothing funny about that.

> I do think I am objective about it, and I do think I'm small-er than I have been before. But when I see other people, maybe because I'm running and going to yoga, everyone is thinner than me. It's the unfairness thing that gets to me,

because I do exercise a lot. I am very conscious of what I eat, and I don't know, whatever I am doing is not enough. I think I have perspective on what a size 6 is. It sounds silly, but I see myself and I know I'm definitely not that thin. Maybe I shouldn't focus on it being unfair that I run. I don't really want to be running, but I am; I think I deserve to be thinner than I am and it's frustrating.

Maybe it's just surprising how relevant it is, it shows how significant it is, how significant an experience it was to be a larger kid and how significant it still is now. I think people see me now and they don't even believe my size was an issue, and that it shouldn't be an issue now. I feel like I shouldn't care about being smaller than other people, and I feel bad that I care about it.

When I have gone to a therapist and talked about my size they act like I am not large now and that it was something in the past. They tell me to go easy on myself, give myself a break. I don't feel like that many people understand, not that many people have had that experience. I mean there must be people who were larger when they were kids, obviously there were, but I don't know them now. I don't know how to identify them now. Just because of what someone looks like now, doesn't tell you what their experiences were like as a kid.

I guess I think there is some value in just talking about it. I guess it's sort of flattering that someone wants to talk to me about it. I never talk about it to anyone. Most people don't realize how emotional they will be talking about it. There's a lot of secrecy and shame. I don't think kids should diet, but growing up fat is really hard.

No, not funny.

22

THE DYNAMIC DUO

One might imagine that in their spare time mother-and-daughter team Cathy and Anna don capes and solve crimes. A modern-day dynamic duo, these two women only stray from a serious mission for the essential pit stops—like to push each other off a curb and giggle like schoolgirls.

Perhaps they don't literally fly, but if they could, it wouldn't be all that surprising. They clearly leap tall buildings. Truth be told, they might make any other mother and daughter team a little jealous—not so much for their powers of strength, but for their ease of camaraderie. To envision them as comic-book heroes hardly seems like an exaggeration, when a mom and a fifteen-year-old daughter not only like each other this much, but also protect each other the way that they do.

Not actually caped crusaders, what makes them so super is even more extraordinary: They, almost like fictional characters, exemplify a functional family.

Cathy, the mom, grew up as a fat kid, although as seems to be common enough, the pictures of her back then don't reflect a kid who was actually fat. She was curvier than other people her age, though not so much fat. That didn't stop her from believing she was fat. Perception is reality, after all. In one of those pictures, she is with her younger siblings—the three were ages nine, ten, and eleven. It being summer time, her kid brother and sister were wearing shorts and tank tops. Cathy had on a long-sleeve shirt buttoned all the way to the top and pants almost to her knees. No one wants to see the skin of a fat kid, or perhaps more essentially, she didn't want anyone to see her fat-kid skin. Her mom claims Cathy was only put on a diet for part of a year during junior high. Cathy remembers always being on a diet, so it must have been one seriously long year. Or, part of a year in junior high is all it takes to get the ball rolling, and from then on you don't need to be put on a diet by anyone else—a child becomes exceedingly self-sufficient at dieting.

Later on, Cathy was supported by her mother in dieting. Even during financially strapped times her mom would gladly write a check to Weight Watchers or Jenny Craig, or whoever was going to help her daughter be slender and beautiful, because she loved her. Cathy's mom did love her, and her intentions were good. She didn't want Cathy to be teased; she wanted her to fit in, to find someone to love her and to have all the things skinny girls get, and fat girls don't. But as they say, the road to hell is paved with good intentions, and that road is a particularly straight shot when it comes to diets.

At the risk of being obvious, and redundant, it's not an overstatement to say Cathy developed a strong hatred of her own body, a pattern of weight loss and gain, and a host of disordered eating problems. Luckily Cathy had a good enough sense of perspective to realize that this pattern was probably not best to repeat, and though she couldn't divert her own childhood, she would never send a child of her own down that road. And she didn't.

Anna is now fifteen, a volatile age in so many ways. But you wouldn't know it from Anna. Perhaps that is because, at least in part, she has been surrounded by beautiful large women—in life, in pictures, in sculptures, and in any way an image can be portrayed that would counter the condemnation for that which is not the singular beauty exalted in a fifteen-year-old girl's life. To teach a girl that her worth is not based on her smallness is a superhuman task, just one more reason this duo have clearly earned their capes.

Cathy's father-in-law spent about a decade before his death living in her home. This was obviously a good portion of Anna's life, and an essential time in terms of building her self-image. Cathy's father-in-law was not quite as, let's say, progressive about the beauty of larger forms, including his own, which would fluctuate greatly in those last years. When large, he would refer to himself as being "a quarter of a ton." For those of us math-challenged and Google-lazy, that is 500 pounds. Now, there certainly are people who weigh a quarter of a ton, though Cathy's father was not one of them; but that is not really the point. It's much more about feeling like a quarter of a ton, and being something worthy of derision.

Cathy spent nearly forty years of her life working on not judging herself by saying things like "I'm a quarter of a ton." She estimates she is able to avoid such self-contempt about 90 percent of the time—after forty years of working on it. Her goal with Anna was to have her at 90 percent from day one. She tried to convince her father-in-law that he didn't deserve his own scorn for illness, weight fluctuations, or for a large body regardless of the reason. The house rule: He wasn't allowed to disparage his body, but if he felt the need, it had to be done in the privacy of his own room. There are some things that are not for the eyes and ears of children.

When Anna's cousin, Cathy's niece, was seven, her mother found her in front of the mirror patting her very fat belly and mocking it, as if her belly's being fat had proved itself bad. Cathy's sister is quite thin, a size 8, as compared to Cathy's size 26. When Cathy's sister gets stressed, she goes down to a 6. Cathy, on the other hand, ends up a 30. We aren't all alike. Anyhow, confused by this behavior, Cathy's sister asked her why her young daughter would have such an attitude toward her little-girl paunch. When Cathy's sister admitted to critical mirror behavior herself, she had her answer. Cathy tries very hard not to do anything of that nature in front of Anna, and now at fifteen, Anna is sure to let her know if she slips up. They do that for each other, but understandably, Anna, not needing a forty-year recovery period from damaged self-image, slips up a lot less.

Cathy, having been subjected to diets prescribed by her parents at an early age, although not approving, is sympathetic to the parents' plight. Parents put their kids on diets out of love, of course.

Interestingly, Anna is far less tolerant on this subject. She does not seem clouded by social convention or compassion for good people who make bad decisions. "My mom says that parents put their kids on diets out of love. I personally think it's out of hatred for their child's body." Harsh. "I know they don't want them to get bullied, or put down, or made fun of, but with the mindset of putting kids on diets, what they are really saying is, 'To protect you, we have to fix you. We need to get rid of that body; you can't have that body.' That is hatred of a fat body." Out of the mouths of babes. She kind of has a point, though. It's easy for a fifteen-year-old to judge, but that doesn't make her wrong.

All right smarty-pants, what should a parent do if their kid gets teased, or to prevent teasing? Teasing does suck. "I think they should be more supportive of their child, and their child's eating habits and exercise. The children that tease, they do it because either they are being bullied themselves, or their parents are bullies to their coworkers; they see this behavior and think it's right. They are modeling poor behavior, or they are having trouble at home—there is always going to be something linked. Either it is imitation or needing to release anger."

Well, that's an explanation, not a resolution. "Someone called my friend ugly and they were hurt. I said, 'Well, you're not ugly. As long as you believe that you are beautiful no one else can tell you otherwise.' As long as the kid knows they are awesome the way they are and totally believes it, no one can make them feel differently. Parents need to reinforce that." Anna is an idealist, perhaps. Maybe she's a bit optimistic. But she has reason to be. Anna speaks from personal experience. This isn't a grown-up telling a child about sticks and stone, it's a fat kid who was raised to think she is remarkable and totally believes it. Perception is reality, remember?

Understanding motivation is one of the most effective ways adults deal with difficult people. Don't let the bastards get you down, and start at an early age. While a parent wanting a kid to diet to protect them from bullying isn't unreasonable, there is a pretty good argument that not buying into the bully is a whole lot more rational, and doable, than changing yourself as protection. How many afterschool specials about not giving the bully our lunch money do we have to see to be able to extrapolate that lunch money is only an analogy for justice? If you're Anna, not many.

It's really the same for societal messages, from Anna's perspective.

> Let's say you have the best-intentioned parent who has good skills; she can't protect her child from fashion magazines or pop stars, or other parents. You can't shield a child from the world unless you completely isolate them in a little plastic bubble. You're never going to be able to shield them from stuff like "easy, breezy CoverGirl." If you were going to, you might as well be a caveman. You can't, you just have to reinforce confidence. I see pictures in magazines of models and they are super thin, and when I look really closely, I notice they are Photoshopped. But I pay attention to details. I see ads all the time that are demeaning and can be very hurtful, like liposuction and Weight Watchers commercials. There was one for losing weight eating one shake a day, that's all you are eating a day. I don't know how another kid would see it, but to me it's just another commercial. Again, you can't shield them, it really has to do with reinforcing confidence.

> People come to me to talk and they're just downing themselves in front of everyone. I tell them to look in the mirror and tell themselves every single morning that they are awesome, that they should look themselves right in the eye, and by next week, they're a lot more confident themselves. So the key is confidence-building with your child, and even the parents can do this themselves. The parents might not be so confident that they are doing a good job in making sure that the child is safe and protected. They can't do it a hundred percent, never, never, ever. Kids see all kinds of things, it's just what happens.

Anna is very well adjusted. Perhaps more well adjusted than most adults, but it's not like she is never challenged. When Anna was twelve, she first got her period, and it lasted for eight weeks. In the beginning, Anna and her mom were excited at this new stage of life; Anna was becoming a woman. But the excitement turned to anxiety and worry, particularly for Anna, who was new to this world, and in her mind it seemed as though she were menstruating to death. First a trip to her pediatrician, who felt this was probably normal enough but considered a gynecologist might be in order. It started out as a formality—the nurse asked routine questions, and the plan was for the doctor to drop in and write a prescription. This was at Planned Parenthood. Cathy thought every girl should know of their local Planned Parenthood, as Mom is not always around. The fact that the doctor was at Planned Parenthood is only really relevant because they should set the bar for respectful and insightful treatment of young women, right?

The doctor walks in, hands Anna the script, gives the basics on how to use it, and says, for no clinically related reason, "You need to lose weight." Neither Anna nor Cathy, sitting right beside her, was expecting this. Cathy, protective and on the defensive, informs the doc that Anna eats well, exercises, and takes dance lessons, and "I am not concerned with her weight at this time, thank you." The doctor left the room. Cathy looks over to Anna for a sign of approval, and gets a high five. Well done, dynamic duo. Except as much as Anna has been taught to feel confident in her skin, and as much as Cathy has learned how to respond to unwanted and unneeded body critiques, we live in the culture we live in, and when it comes to fat, we are fragile.

In retrospect, Anna has no recollection of her mother even being in the room. As she remembers it, her mom left before the doctor got there—which is not possible, because Cathy is clear on the details of the exchange and knows she never left the room. Anna, it seems, was traumatized enough by what felt like an assault, that she had complete tunnel vision. She was paralyzed by this authority figure, whose job it is heal and do no harm, but who instead matter-of-factly, but not without judgment, supported all of society's condemnations and countered her mother's supportive teachings in a shocking split second. It actually took Anna some consideration to realize and admit that she was hurt. She is used to being a pillar of strength, but Anna is a person, not a pillar.

> I do not really remember how I felt. I realize that a lot of times, pretty much everyone will block out a situation that was horribly stressful and hurtful—for example the death of a loved one or abuse when you were a child. Everyone has that wall in their brain, no matter how tall it is or what is behind it. I do remember it was a bright room. Mom was wearing a black shirt. I was probably wearing a uniform because it was after school.

Cathy remarks how Anna likens the experience to child abuse or death of a loved one. Duly noted. Even with someone as well adjusted and protected as Anna, people are volatile around this issue, and it doesn't take much to cause trauma. Now, in fairness, Anna didn't instantaneously head into a tailspin or spiral out of control. Anna, being Anna, picked herself up and moved on. She didn't develop an eating disorder or become obsessed with every inch of fat. But not everyone is as well adjusted and protected as Anna.

Cathy isn't immune either. This wasn't her first rodeo. She had had "the conversation" with Anna's pediatrician before, and during the first one, she cried the entire time. Composure against condemnation is a skill, and practice makes, well, someone better at it than they were before.

Of course this was not Anna's first experience contending with unwanted "advice," either. Once, when she was around age eleven and minding her own business, sitting on her front lawn playing the guitar, some clever dude drove by and yelled out the window, "Lose some weight, fat ass." A drive-by insult. It was more surprising to Anna than anything. She went running into the house, incredulous. "Mom, you are not going to believe what this guy said to me!" And she was given a pass for calling him a dick. Facts are facts.

What Cathy found most interesting about the experience was how differently her daughter responded than she herself would have at that age. "If that had happened to me at eleven, I wouldn't have told a soul; and I would have run right up to my room, hidden in the closet, and eaten a bag of candy. I couldn't tell my mom; I was too afraid she would say he had a point." Whatever one might think of fat children, that right there illustrates the difference between raising a child who will, or won't, end up with an eating disorder.

At Anna's grandmother's house there is a massive jar—grandmother's cookie jar. When Anna and her cousin would visit, inevitably they would ask for a cookie. Anna was seven. Anna's cousin would ask for another and her grandmother would respond, "Of course, dear." Fifteen minutes later, Anna asked for another—she had eaten only one, and her cousin had already had two. Her grandmother would respond, "I'm sorry, I think you've had enough." Though Anna was polite to this and young enough not to say it out loud, her response was "WTF?!" She didn't even know exactly what WTF meant, but she understood the sentiment. WTF?

It was the same at her aunt's. They had a thing for Oreos there, and you could always count on an Oreo in the pantry. Anna would ask for one, because what little kid wouldn't? "Didn't you already have one?" "No." It was just assumed. Anna was a fat kid, and fat kids must have already gotten their pudgy little fingers on the Oreos, somehow. What Anna remembers most about this treatment, aside from how unjust it seemed, was that the focus wasn't on how lovely their little granddaughter or niece was, but on her weight and what she was eating. WTF? How is a kid supposed to make sense of this? It seemed punitive, and it was, and her crime was having more fat on her body.

In truth, in retrospect, Anna isn't certain how often this actually happened. She knows her grandmother had put her mom on diets as a child, so her behavior made sense. Her aunt, though, is a nurse, a health enthusiast, and very knowledgeable. She knows about the smart ways to feed children. What Anna is remembering, more than anything else, is how it felt. It felt penalizing and she remembers that, even if perhaps it didn't happen exactly how she describes it. At Anna's own house they don't have cookies. They are allowed to have cookies, but history has shown that a bag will get eaten in a night, and everyone will feel sick as a result, so they go over to Cathy's sister's for their cookie fix, or just buy what they want when they want it.

They try to eat using the rules of "intuitive eating," recognizing what your body needs and when you are full or actually hungry. This may be a bit easier for Anna than Cathy. Cathy wasn't raised like this and spent many years dieting. She also spent many years recovering, so it takes a real effort. Recognizing that desiring a cookie is probably more about taste than hunger isn't always easy, especially because cookies just taste so good. That's the point of cookies. So they support each other in this. Not to avoid cookies, but to recognize what it is the body is craving, and to satisfy that need, even if it's just to have something that tastes so good. It's a subtle difference, but one Cathy believes is very important, and Anna has been raised to understand.

This is what they find so troubling about what's going on with the "childhood-obesity epidemic." They are both quite politically minded about it. Health is measurable, but not by weight. Some children eat in a healthy way and exercise and are still bigger, and others barely eat at all, or make poor choices when they do, but because they look thin, they are assumed to be healthy. When this is the case, neither child is probably getting the best messages, or care. It's the focus on fat rather than health. Our society seems hell-bent on it.

When the Michelle Obama Let's Move! campaign began, Cathy and Anna were open-minded. They were thrilled to see the community gardens and the focus on fun exercise and learning about nutrition. "There are so many awesome ideas in it, so many awesome things they are doing; in fact, almost everything they started doing was great. But then it changed from a campaign about health to eliminating childhood obesity for the next generation.

I find it hard to believe that's even possible. Nature is so diverse, naturally diverse, there are many shapes and sizes of everything. That's how it's misguided, how it's labeled." Anna is quick to chime in about why the focus went from health to weight: money. Cathy agrees. "There is not much money in growing vegetables in your backyard or walking around the block. There has to be money made somewhere, and there is money in the obesity epidemic. It's unfortunate, because it ruins a great idea."

As far as obesity in children goes, Cathy and Anna are pretty consistent with their beliefs, and as a duo respond together:

> If you mean a diet where calories are counted and every meal is planned around weight loss, no kid should be on that kind of diet. Any person's diet can be adjusted so that it's filled with nutrients and not junk. That's the first step in seeing the reality of the situation. If you want the child to be healthy regardless of what size the body is, you look at what they have access to, their home environment, how much exercise they get, how much stress is put on them daily. If you move in healthier directions with all that, specific to the child, that child will be healthier. They may become smaller or they may stay the same size. If their body is not functioning well and that is causing them to keep on extra weight, that weight will probably go away with changes. But you have to be focused on the health, not the weight. You also have to look at the bigger surroundings of the child—society doesn't realize they are often making the surroundings worse, and influencing how the parents think of the child and how the child thinks of herself. It's a multidimensional issue.

What Anna has learned from her peers is that conventional stereotypes are just not true. Her friends are all over the map in terms of what they eat, how much they exercise, and what they weigh. They are also very diverse in terms of how they feel about themselves. One male friend is in a continual state of angst, worried that he will never find a girlfriend. He feels that no one will like him because he is fat. The thing is, he's not even particularly fat. He just thinks he is, and his issues with girls seem, to Anna at least, to be more about attitude than appearance. It's not just a female problem anymore. Society seems to be leveling the playing field in terms of fat anxiety.

On the other hand, Anna is not particularly interested in dating. It just isn't her primary focus as a fifteen-year-old. She prefers to concern herself with school and dance class, the plays she is in, and her own brand of political activism. Ironic, since she has already been in three relationships, though her first was at age nine, so she's not sure it counts. She has been involved with a boy for six months now, but she doesn't worry about it one way or the other. "I wouldn't just focus everything on one person. That's unhealthy in general. Focusing on one thing to the point where if it doesn't happen it seems like it will completely crush your life forever, it's not healthy for your eating habits or your grades. I knew a person whose grades dropped because she was so obsessed with someone." That is just not her style.

Her self-esteem is good enough that she has perspective on whatever happens. "That's about right. Occasionally when I first introduce myself to people, I get the once-over, the judgmental once-over, like the 'Is that really who I'm about to talk to?' once-over. But in my mind, I just roll my eyes and go on with what we're supposed to be doing. I feel confident in myself and people see that confidence is about more than size. I think the confidence is bigger than my weight."

If that isn't representative of a modern-day superhero, what is?

23

DIGGING YOUR GRAVE WITH YOUR FORK, AND OTHER THINGS TO DO FOR AT LEAST SEVEN DECADES

An Interview with Daniel Pinkwater

Born in 1942, Daniel Pinkwater is the author and sometimes illustrator of over 80 (and counting) wildly popular books. He is currently an occasional commentator on National Public Radio's *All Things Considered* and *Car Talk*, and appears regularly on *Weekend Edition Saturday*, where he reviews exceptional kids' books with host Scott Simon. He has, in the past, had his own show on NPR. Frankly, his bio is just too long to do justice here.

Many of his books include fat characters, though they are mostly incidentally fat. He has written about fat as a theme. He is fat. He was a fat kid.

He is also charming, brilliant, witty, prolific, and one of the most interesting and entertaining people you would ever have the pleasure to speak with. Daniel Pinkwater in his own words:

Q: Tell me about being fat as a child.

I am looking at a class photo taken at the Nettelhorst School in Chicago on October 27, 1948. I was in the third grade. There are approximately forty kids in the class; that's how they were in those days. I'm going to count now—seven fat children out of the class of forty. I am seated cross-legged on the floor, with a fat kid on either side.

We all look good.

That's my statement.

Oh, maybe there are eight. This one, I'm going to count her as fat, I'm pretty sure this girl grew up to be fat. Wait a minute, nine—this little short girl is fat. I remember her. So nine out of forty kids in 1948 were markedly fat, clearly fat. Fat would be one of the terms you would use to describe them if you weren't afraid to say fat, and nobody was then.

Q: Does that seem like a lot?

It doesn't seem like a lot or a little. I'm just stating a fact. I have the earliest documentary evidence of me in society as a fat kid. Of the three fat boys in the front row, of which I am one, all of us have neckties. Only one other boy in the picture is wearing a necktie—he's a lawyer now. But no other boy is wearing a necktie. Also, two of the three fat kids sitting together have a button on their lapel, which I think indicates they are members of the student council. It was Chicago and so it may be that we presented an appearance that related to, or associated with, prominence or importance, particularly in politics. There wasn't a universal health scare about being fat yet.

Q: Did people discuss your being fat?

I cannot actually recall, and I will not extrapolate or interpolate any particular attention paid to the fact of being fat. It wasn't a particular factor. There were so many other markers. There were kids in the third grade that still occasionally had a peeing in the pants accident. One of the fat girls was a kissing bug; she kissed every boy in the whole class. And many of them were refugees and immigrants. It was right after the war, so some of them were escapees, war-shocked children from Europe. Many of the kids in this picture had parents who didn't speak much English, or any. There was plenty going on; fat didn't come into it.

Q: How did you feel about being fat?

Fat was handy on the playground when it came to throwing a punch. I could put a little more behind a punch than a thinner kid, and so those few conflicts that arose—and I'd like to state for the record that I never started one of them—I could finish them pretty good. And also you could sit upon or fall upon someone. So you could use weight in fighting effectively. So it was a plus, and also it meant that some people might gravitate to one such as me for protection, because nobody would start with me, because I could put them away.

There was a fair amount of fighting—it was Chicago, it was a city school, it was not a cheerful, happy, sunshiny place. The playground's entire surface was gravel, so when you went down you went down on gravel. At the very least, your knees would get hurt. I'm sure the adults who designed it said good enough for them, gravel will help them mature and learn about reality, build character.

I think I was moderately popular. In the picture, I have a rather serious look. I think I am the only kid—here's something that was probably of much more interest—I am the only one with glasses in the whole forty. Probably not the only one who needed them, but I had them.

Q: What did your parents do?

My father was not a gangster. He had given that up. And, my mother was not a prostitute, or a gangster's whore. She had given that up. They were respectable citizens doing their best. They made a good living (in the black market). I would say that half the kids in the class were middle-class children, but I just think that the only reason I had glasses was I couldn't see the black-board so I acted out and was a problem, and some smart person worked out that I couldn't read the stuff so I was amusing myself by behaving badly.

Q: Did you ever get teased for being fat?

I do not remember ever being teased for being fat, unless you count an instance that struck me as so unique that I remember it clearly. My mother took to taking me to the doctor, my parents loved going to doctors, so I got dragged along, and of course the doctor identified me as fat and gave my mother a little lecture on how that was wrong—and we did this many times with more than one doctor—and he would give her a printed-out diet to put me on, you know a half of grapefruit and a half a slice of toast, and so forth.

Then the doctor would give me a lollipop which always struck me as bizarre even then at that age—here he's just made a speech about how I shouldn't be fat and he's told my mother not to let me have sweets and he's given her this preposterous diet on paper to put me on, and then he gives me a candy.

What's wrong with that picture?

So he gives me the sucker, and after she would take me to a restaurant downtown and allow me to order a meal of my favor-ite things, because I was going to have to go on a diet, poor child. Then we would go home and the diet would last, maximally, a day. She would give me the prescribed diet food on the first day and the second day it was forgotten. She didn't like to prepare it, it didn't look like I was enjoying it, she was making bacon and eggs for everyone else, and I got it too.

Here's the thing I was working up to telling you. On one of these doctor visits, just about this age, just about eight. There I am at the pediatrician's in my underwear, having been examined and possibly having blood drawn, and weighed and all the different stuff. And I'm in the little room where the doctor examines you, and another kid, also in his undies, comes into the room, and he says, "Fatty, fatty, I lost 8 pounds, why can't you?" And he runs out. I assume to be given his lollipop reward by the doctor.

It was clear to me that the doctor had put him up to it, to inspire me. Here's the thing about me: I was born very intelligent, really smart, it's been wearing off for a lifetime, to where I am now, but at that point this brain was fresh and it just worked like a charm, so my instant response was what would be the mature response, I believe, which was: What a tacky thing to do! And then thinking, how does the kid feel being put up to it, the successful eight-pound-loser, and what does this doctor got in his mind?

But I was already somewhat hip because, I don't know if you have been to doctors a lot in your life, but there tend to be catchphrases that go around. If you're seeing several doctors in a short period, you'll discover them all saying the same formulaic things. And in this case, every doctor I was taken to told me, "You'll be dead by the time you're forty." This upset my mother more than it upset me because that seemed like a ripe old age.

It stayed with me, though, and I was very surprised at the age of forty when I didn't die.

And then I realized that this was what your Scientologists call an engram, that had been lurking in there the whole time—it was errant nonsense. How could they predict such a thing? But I'd never bothered to refute it, I'd never bothered to dismiss it. And so it was just there as a given because I hadn't questioned it. Forty-one, forty-two, I still wasn't dead, seventy-one I'm still not dead, and as soon as I realized for sure that this was malarkey, which I would have realized immediately if I'd thought about it even, I felt very liberated.

Q: When did you come to the realization that you probably weren't going to drop dead in the way the doctors predicted?

When did I realize I wasn't going to die at forty? When I didn't die at forty. I hadn't really thought about it ever since, except I do remember that they all said it. They'd say, "You're digging your grave with your fork and you'll be dead by the time you're forty." I knew enough to ignore adults, but I didn't bother to question them.

Also I had, as I'd intimated, a highly dysfunctional, fucked-up family. So I learned very early what they were doing, and therefore, by extrapolation, that maybe most adults don't know as much as they pretend to. If I wasn't so very bright as a child this might have made me insecure, but I was like eh, there's many interesting things, and this wasn't one of them. So I went about my business, and I think that sums up my whole experience being a fat child. It was an interesting world. I lived in an interesting place. There were lots of things going on. It was a rich environment. Not that anyone set out to make it so, it just was. Being fat wasn't interesting.

Q: What was so interesting that it distracted you from being fat?

In the backyards, the kids would play out the plots of classic literature and also famous battles. There were a number of kids, and we played Gettysburg and Bunker Hill and Iwo Jima, and also the Three Musketeers and the Hunchback of Notre Dame, from the classic comic. The older kids would always act as the directors and the little kids would be the extras. We would work from the actual text. And this prompted me to bear down on learning to read, because I wanted to read these stories myself, and I even once got to play Quasimodo. I went up on the back porch and held Ruthie, the little girl from downstairs, over my head and hollered, "Sanctuary, sanctuary." So, it was, and then there was a lot of cultural confluence, it was just an interesting place to be, there was a lot of stuff going on.

I had siblings who taught me things. I lived in an apartment house of four stories and a basement apartment and there was one just like it next to it, separated by a driveway to an old-fashioned backyard, and old-fashioned garages where you used to put your Model T. In those two buildings, three kids growing up at the same time grew up to be children's authors, go figure.

So I didn't sit around thinking about being fat because there was much going on, and nobody cared, except the doctor who was threatening me with an early death (only it didn't seem early), and my mother, who was conscientious enough to put me on the diet for a day. And beyond that, it wasn't an issue.

Q: Your parents weren't concerned you were fat?

They were neglectful parents, the best thing you can have. Nothing is better. My father could barely read English, or any language, I think. It took him two hours to struggle through the newspaper. This meant that any book I read he hadn't read. This put me ahead of him in some ways. I never met kids different from me until I got to college; they had been exposed to all the finer things all along, but they didn't seem to really value them: "Oh yes, *Moby Dick*, we had that in our junior year in prep school." "Well aren't you excited?" "No, it's a good story. And I know some things to say about it to get me an A on the test." "Yeah but, but didn't it drive you crazy how great it is?" "You're so naive."

Please, when I'm born next time, let me be born again to a rough ex-gangster immigrant who can't read English, and let me be naive. I want to realize the greatness of *Moby Dick*.

Q: Was your mother worried about you dying young?

She was worried about what she was going to buy in Marshall Field's department store before we went home. She was going through the motions of being a normal wife and mother. She even pretended that she graduated from high school, to the point of having various mementos of high school around, like a book called *The Girl Graduates Book*—it was an all-purpose nonspecific yearbook for someone to fake they went to high school. She was trying to fit into the middle-class and be a regular American. And she was, actually. She didn't really retain things in her head unless they pertained to her, and those things weren't too deep. Benign neglect. I love it.

Q: Were any of your siblings fat?

All of them, except my sister. My sister is very fat now, but she looked like Ingrid Bergman in those days, which was cool for her because she was a girl.

Q: Were your parents fat?

No. Not at all.

Q: So where to do you think the fatness comes from?

I think it comes from the angels. Is there a genetic route there? Who knows? It's not uncommon for all the children in a family to be fat and the parents not. I guess we could work out some reasons, but I'm not one of your scientists or academics on this topic. Various things occur to one, but why waste time thinking about it?

I do want to make a statement, which relates a little bit about what I've been telling you up until now, which is this: All my concerns with being fat, and becoming thin, which I've done a couple of times, have been by way of other people's concerns, wishes, or demands. Never my own. It never bothered me, it never entered my mind. It wasn't interesting to me, just because, the only opprobrium that stung me a little was when it was suggested I was lazy or weak or incapable or undisciplined. So to prove a point, I lost 100 pounds a couple times. But not just on my own, but when somebody challenged me or wanted me to very much.

Like my father-in-law, when I wanted to marry my wife, I had to do the old-fashioned asking for her hand, and seeing if he could make me drunk, which he tried to do with lots of good whisky. And here's a dignified guy and he said, "The only concern I have is your weight and that's because I'm concerned about your health. I love my daughter, and I don't want him dying when he's forty." Ah geez, this again. "Will you promise me to make a special effort to lose weight if you can?" Yes, I promise, and I did. I gained it back, but I did do it.

Q: Were you ever traumatized in any way by being fat?

Yes, once. I've always been attracted to hiking and mountaineering, of a mild nature, not with ropes and peptones, but I like scrambling up things. I was quite a strong, athletic young man. I was walking by myself on the bluffs, on the Palisades right across from New York, which has some wild country. Right across from Yonkers you get into some pretty interesting woods and stuff. And I had my little knapsack and my boots and I was just having a good time hiking in the woods, which I used to do all the time. And I took a path I'd never taken along the top of these cliffs of about 450 feet high over the Hudson. It was a path leading somewhat downward toward the river. Making my way down the cliff face in a way, but gradually in the woods, I came upon a sign that said "Danger, don't go beyond this point."

It looked like an old sign. It was weathered and almost illegible. And I thought, this can't be, Boy Scouts put it up in the 1930s, I'm gonna keep going. And I found myself getting down into a...I found a path I didn't know existed that ran above and parallel to the Hudson River. And I said, I can take this path back and surely there's a way to get to the top of the cliff and I'll find my way to the place where I left my car. Having a great old time, and then there was a little bit of a rocky area, there had been a little bit of a rock-slide. "That must be what the sign was about, I'll just traverse this rock-slide." Well, it was a much bigger rock-slide than I had thought, no one knew where I was, I hadn't told anyone I was going. And I'm clambering over these rocks, which get bigger and bigger, and big as a house, and now I have to decide do I want to turn back and go all the way back? "This can't last much longer, I'll bet ya." I come off the side of this and basically it was a kind of scalloped shore, so you couldn't see down the river along this rock-slide. And I always thought, just as I get around this it will be over and there will be a way to continue, the path with continue.

Well it didn't, and it got to be a huge deal, and now I'm doing things I read about in a book that mountain climbers do, where you're putting your back against one, it's called a chimney, there's sort of a fissure or a space, and you put your back against one rock and your feet against the other and you walk up, you work your way up this thing. This is getting to be a little crazy for a 300-pounder. And then some of these rocks are unstable. I have a stick with me and I'm poking them and they rock and I have to decide where to put my feet, and there are these deep pitfalls with brackish river water at the bottom that clearly fill up when the tide comes in. And I say, if I fall down there it will be 100 years before anybody finds my bones, what the hell am I doing here? I'm not suited for this kind of climbing.

And I got across that, and I did feel severely chagrined and embarrassed by my weight. I came off the thing, obviously. It was very interesting because the little piece of forest I came into hadn't been visited for a long time—hikers didn't come that way, and the little animals were very tame, they weren't afraid of me. They came up to me like a Disney movie, so like bunnies and chipmunks and birds and things hopping around my feet as I walked along. And sure enough I found what amounted to a stairway cut into the cliff and I got up and got back to my car and was very sore the next day.

Q: Did you respond to that embarrassment in any way?

Yes, I blamed my brother. It was really rough going, I had gotten in trouble, and I had done a very foolish thing, and I was in real danger. And I was talking out loud and I was talking to him, and I was saying, "It's you, you son of a bitch," with all the adventure stories and men's magazines of the times, which were all about daring and expeditioning that influenced me to try a thing like this, "You jerk, it's your fault." It turns out I wasn't too fat to be a daredevil, it just wasn't so pleasant. I was embarrassed that I got into it. I was grateful that I got out of it, and also I think the reason the animals all came up to me may not have been that they were unaccustomed to people, but that I had spent—maybe that's why people do things like this—I had spent all of my aggression and anger and tears and dangerousness on the rocks, and when I came off the rocks and was in a safe environment. I was completely Christlike to the little animals. They knew they had nothing to fear because there was nothing; I wasn't going to eat them or hurt them or anything. It had all been purged out of me. That's maybe why people climb mountains, they spend all of their unwanted or unnecessary energy on the mountain—they spend all that negative stuff. And when they get to the top they feel close to God? I don't know.

Q: In school was there physical fitness stuff?

I could not climb those ropes, I simply couldn't. But by that time all kinds of other questionable features of my personality had flowered. I was a habitual truant and I would refuse to go to school and I would come in late and they didn't know what to do with me. And also, I would complain of being tired, because I claimed to be an insomniac. The truth is I had a Hallicrafter shortwave radio and I stayed up very late at night listening to the shortwave broadcasts. So they put me in a kind of remedial gym class for people with mental or physical problems, or whatever. And this was great because there was no rope-climbing, and they would let us take naps. "This is a matter of health and you're obviously tired, so you just lie down on the mat and take a nap." Fine by me, coach. Did they blame it on my fatness? I don't know that they did.

I had a friend in high school that was fat like me, a lovely guy, only died the other year. When I met him I was sitting in the back row of Mrs. McMillan's English class in Lake View High School in Chicago. Mrs. McMillan was an enthusiastic anti-Semite, and in those days you could be one. She used to make a set speech to her classes every year when school began, about how there are some people who do not want us to have a fine country and who want to destroy everything that is good, and who are evil and corrupt, and those people, children, are the Jews. They're very clever and sneaky and they're everywhere, and you must always be aware of them and beware of them.

We loved Mrs. McMillan, and here's something that will possibly inform you as to why I didn't have any problems with being teased. In this school, which was in a German neighborhood in Chicago, and very few of the kids were Jewish, every kid who drew Mrs. McMillan for English would acquire, if they weren't Jewish and had one, a Star of David or a mezuzah and wear it around their neck outside their clothes on the first day of class. Every single one of them. And as she gave her anti-Semitic speech she would start to focus on the fact that every kid had a little Jewish symbol hanging around his or her neck, and it would be fun to watch the sickening expression on her face.

There was also a kid in the school who was interested in politics—he was also the first-out gay I ever met. This was like 1956 or 7, told everybody he was gay, and what's more, he didn't have to tell ya, you would have guessed it immediately. He had beautiful skin, he had gorgeous golden hair, he had the bluest of eyes, and teeth like pearls. And the first time I met him, he said, "I am a homosexual," and I said, it would be a shame if you were anything else. Well, he was interested in student politics and he ran for student office all the time. He never got elected because he gave a lousy speech, but I never heard anybody make a remark about him being gay, ever. Ever.

And the kids all by themselves, defied Mrs. McMillan.

So I'm sitting in the back by myself and this kid comes in late and he's carrying a whole bunch of books and a pair of drumsticks, that you play drums with, not from a chicken. And he comes in and he's disheveled-looking and he's sweaty and confused and his clothes are awry, and he trips as he comes in and he falls down with an enormous clatter, dropping the books, and the drumsticks clattering on the ground, and he's just about my size. And I think, oh look, the poor kid is slow, I'll be nice to him, he can sit by me.

This is my friend Bob, it turns out the falling was a deliberate thing. He had taken some wrestling lessons and he could do a number of great falls, and one of the falls he could do was like a professional wrestler's fall where you go up in the air and you appear to land right on your spine. But really what you do is break the fall by bending your knees and landing on the soles of your feet and hit the ground, and in effect, ease yourself down so you don't really fall on your back and break it. And we would meet in the hall and we would circle around each other and sort of grapple for a second and I would pretend to flip him, but actually under his own power he would go up in the air, do a full summersault forward, and then fall on his back. Pretty good for a kid in the high 200s.

Okay, he was a gambler, he made his living as a gambler later in life, and he always was trying to lose weight, all through his life, and with the usual results. And the last time I saw him was a couple of years ago, and we had a meal in the diner and he frightened me by what he ate, and when we left he said you're not fat, and I said yes I am. He said no, you're not fat. I said what do you weigh. He said 365. I said I was at the doctor last week; I weigh 395. No you don't, you're not even fat. I'll take you with me, his office is right over here, he's got one of those electronic scales and they'll let me use it, I'll show you, 395. But you're not fat. How can you say it Bob? I'm 395, I'm fatter than you, I'm your height. But you're not fat.

On a deep level I never thought I was. He was picking up the vibe. It just hasn't been interesting to me. I've had no reason to be fat. I am fat, I haven't had any reason to make that an important part of my persona. I had to kick and scream not to be taken into the army. They were going to induct me. And it never occurred to me to say to them, can't you see I'm too fat to be a soldier? Because they weren't seeing it, because I don't see it. It's just not a factor. I'm aware of it. I'm interested in the sociology of it. I've written little pieces, which brought you to me, about it. But speaking as honestly as I can, it doesn't enter my thoughts, it never has. It hasn't been an impediment because, to me, it's not even there.

Yeah, there's things I obviously can't do, I wouldn't try to traverse that rock-slide again—I climbed Kilimanjaro, but not to the top because, yeah, it would kill me. But that didn't seem big. I've heard there are free-range fat people, a term I've heard from Marilyn Wann. And they are statistically invisible because they're healthy, they go about their business, they're not much concerned, and I guess I'm one of those. I haven't suffered from being a fat child. I didn't want to play tennis, so it didn't matter. If I had a consuming desire to play tennis and couldn't lose weight, that would have been a problem, but it didn't come up.

Q: How did you get interested in writing about fat?

Well, I had this gig with NPR for twenty-five years, and about twenty years of that one program, I had to come up with a little commentary every week. And I had, by way of keeping my word to my father-in-law. I went down to Duke to the famous Rice program, where I did nothing but spend six months with fat people, and just out of boredom I started doing what you're doing, which is interviewing them. But I didn't do it as a formal interview, I would just engage them in conversation, and I got an idea about what they were thinking about and what their experience had been. I recognize completely, especially having been with them, the problems that exist for a lot of people.

But to be honest, they didn't exist for me. I can see where it could have, but it hasn't conflicted with anything important to me. I had a very satisfactory romantic life, I had a successful professional life, I've engaged in all kinds of interesting adventures that I could do. There were things I knew I couldn't do, but that would be true of anyone that's got limitation. And I'm a sort of outward-directed person, I'm not a touchy-feely friendsy person, but I'm interested in what's going on around me, including the other humans. So I'm never bored.

I'm a good artist, I'm a very good writer and these things just— not only did my mother forget all about what my doctor said, I forget about it even before she did. I wasn't home yet, back at our apartment, before I'd totally forgotten and moved on to what I wanted to think. It wasn't important to me. At various times, out of affection or connection to people for whom it was a big deal, like in the case of my father-in-law, I made it my business, and pretended very hard that I was taking it seriously, and even lost weight, a lot of weight. But it just didn't really loom large.

Q: Was there any anger or annoyance about him wanting you to lose weight?

No, because he was like a straight American father, my wife's father, and she loved him and he was a cool guy and I understood where he was coming from. And I wanted him to respect me and be happy that I was coming into the family. No. What's more, he lent me a few dollars to go down there, to Rice. I spent a lot of money in that place.

Q: The other people at that place that you informally interviewed, did they have other perceptions?

I would say that every one of them was reacting to the viewpoint of others, trying to satisfy someone else. None of them, if they had not been put under some kind of pressure from other people, would have ever thought to go and do something as drastic as that. I went because my physician in Hoboken said, "There is only one man who can cure you." By the way, that formula, I have since learned, is a cue to get up and walk away fast. Whenever someone says, "Only I can help you," run. He says there is only one man who can cure you, and I can get you into this program in North Carolina. So I went. I said okay, if this is the only way, I'll do it.

I spent a lot of time with the old Nazi who ran it, Dr. Kempner, who said, "Ya, ven I vas a docta in za camps (he wasn't an inmate, he was a visiting SS physician I guess), I noticed that the people were losing weight." Do tell. "I thought, zis is interesting, because many of za ozer problems vent away." Yeah, especially when they gassed them, right? I used to give him the Hitler salute quite often, and he would always grab you by the upper arm, he'd be feeling for—you can make a quick judgment of someone's body mass index if you feel the fat on their upper arm. He'd say, "Don't do zat! I waz never for him, unt I told him so." This is making me feel great about you, doc.

Q: What was his magic?

He would give people rice. Thrice-washed rice, a half a cup, twice a day. And allow them no salt of any kind. So their electrolytes got out of balance and some of them dropped dead. I mentioned this and he said, "Ya, zey were sick ven zey came, so zey died, ya." I said they died because they have heart problems because they don't have any potassium chloride and sodium. "Ya, itz true, itz a dangerous conditions, za treatment iz extreme, ya, they die." He was a madman.

Q: That's exactly the same perspective as the bariatric surgery now?

Of course, doctors are not nice people. If you meet a doctor who is an ethical person, and I have met a couple, that's quite rare.

Q: Were the other people at the place more emotionally traumatized?

Yes, yeah, it was not a happy crew. Except one guy—while doing the rice diet, the rice diet would certainly work, the same as going into Dachau would have worked—but what he would do is drive over to Greensboro every week and go to Weight Watchers and pretend that he was on their diet. Of course he was losing faster than any of them because he was being starved, systemically starved. But what he was doing was racking up such a great record of a loser that he got to be a lecturer. You make money in Weight Watchers, there's no end to make money off of fat people, so he was feathering his nest for when he got out of the Rice program by becoming a major Weight Watchers lecturer. So he seemed to be happy.

The rest of them were all wretches, they'd be scared to death. Some of them had serious health problems, I don't deny, and I just have to put in a word of sanity, that there can presumably be cases where being fat's a threat to health and then you've got to do something about it or you're going to be sick, or you might die, and those cases, which are not as common as all that in my guesstimation. I haven't looked at the literature in many, many years, but what I read led me to believe, yeah, I run a higher risk of a number of things being a fat person. How much higher? Not much at all. A percentage point? A fraction of a percentage? I'll take those odds. Ask an ethical doctor, if you know one, who is honest and will answer your questions: What do you recommend I do, lose weight or stop smoking? Lose weight or get some exercise? Lose weight or avoid stress? Lose weight or eat healthier foods? Every time he's going to answer the opposite of lose weight. I'm not saying it's bad for you to lose weight, but it's not as high on the list as some of these other things.

So those people who were extremists went there and lost the weight, conceivably, if they could survive the radical starvation diet, and there was fasting as well, although the difference between what they fed you and fasting was really not much. Then at one point I quit Kempner, because how long can you be friends with a Nazi? And I went to a rival program there, where they just put you on a diet. It worked about as well, I lost about 100 pounds and I came back and I was thin. And many of my friends refused to know me. Many of my male friends refused to know me as a nonfat person. They couldn't explain it, they said I don't know you anymore, you're different, I don't want to be around you anymore; you make me nervous.

I've tended to always get along with aggressive A-type people, I don't know why, maybe because my father was one. I get along fine with them, but one of the things that they found attractive about me was that I didn't seem to be a threat. They seemed to think that because I wasn't a threat, I couldn't best them or compete for women. All untrue. But when I wasn't fat, they couldn't rationalize knowing me. Now I seemed scary to them, because they were insecure, I guess.

The other thing when I came back was every time I caught a glimpse of my reflection in a shop window or something, I would be startled, unpleasantly started. I didn't like that. Unless I prepared myself to look in the mirror, I just glimpsed myself with my new contours, I didn't like it. I also found that I was now attractive to a type of woman who would have never been interested in me before and I didn't want their attention. I was attractive to shallow women, and I thought, where do all these bimbos come from? I never knew any women like this. I always knew interesting, nice women.

Q: Did you not like being thin?

Not at all, really.

My story in a nutshell: I'm a happy externally oriented person, very smart in my younger days, who is fat, but didn't want to give it the time or weight, so to speak, to interfere with this beautiful life.

I'm looking at pictures of myself as a little kid. He's a happy child. He's happy by nature. He's a sweet little kid. Then you look at my father and my grandfather, two of the most frightening

Jews ever to walk the earth. Somehow or other, just a genetic fluke, a bright happy child. I drew the personality I got. I was lucky. I wasn't insensitive. I was too amused and interested to buy any of this negative stuff. It didn't stick, it wasn't interesting to me. There was a period where I really wanted to become kind of a dramatic, tragic youth, but I couldn't bring it off. Too many things made me laugh. Just luck.

Q: So you think that those of us who are fat and miserable, we drew the emotional short straw?

In part, that was nature, and then there was nurture. So somebody, instead of saying pull your socks up and have an ice cream and laugh, they said everything that's wrong is because you're fat. And you said, I knew something was wrong, I knew it was my fault. You were caught. But they would have gotten you anyway; fat had nothing to do with it.

I've made my contribution to the struggle by writing funny things about it. Very gratifying to me, I was reading reviews of my most recent novel, and they all say it's about this fat kid. I never say he's fat. I never allude to in the least that he's fat, in the whole book. They are experiencing him as a fat person because they are readers of mine and something I do for my readers who are fat, because a lot of them are, because a lot of people are, especially my readers are, is I'll write a novel of about 300 pages about a kid's experiences and adventures and I'll make one reference to the fact that he's fat, and the reviewer who is fat will always mention it. And finally, the reviewer will mention it even if I haven't.

Q: Why are many of your readers fat, besides a lot of people being fat?

They're smart, they're sedentary, they eat salami while they read.

I'll tell you one more thing. I'll be driving in my car and I'll see some guy waddling down the street, some 350-pound guy, he's progressing along, and I'll catch myself saying damn that's a good-looking guy. I had a lot of girlfriends. They seemed to like me. They seemed to like the look of me, and in the beginning, what do you do with girlfriends, who understands that? But I started to think that it's possible that I'm pleasing to them, and then I'm driving around Poughkeepsie, New York, and I see some fat guy walking along and I say you know, that's a good-looking guy. Damn, he's a good-looking fella.

Q: Why do you like the way fat people look?

Their beautiful, they're round, they move well as a rule, because you've got to be strong, they have a kind of grace. I like elephants too. That was a breakthrough for me because my father's epithet for me was "little elephant," and that got to me, that's the one that got to me. So I went to Africa and I hung out with elephants, and I realized, my God, they're gorgeous, they're majestic, they are wonderful and intelligent and scary. I love them. So that was me working out some of my fat issues. I didn't stress that in the interview because I don't think people should give a lot of importance to that. But I went all the way to Africa and the first reason I wanted to go is that I wanted to visit the elephants, my fellow elephants. They didn't see it that way. They didn't say, "One of us, one of us." They just said, "Schmuck, another tourist, let's scare him."

EPILOGUE

THE WALRUS WAS PAUL

I have two final stories that I will tell, and they represent a progression of my life as a fat-child-to-fat-adult, as best as any stories can. That I am able to tell both of these stories is a direct result of therapy, in which I have engaged a great deal over the years. When I first started, in my early twenties—not counting the time I was forced to attend as a child and told the doctor to fuck off because he looked like Ronald McDonald, and that was the end of that—I was unable to tell these stories to my therapists. In fairness, the second story did not yet exist, but the first seemed too humiliating to share, even in therapy, where humiliating stories are the bread and butter.

Eventually, and I believe it was at least a decade later, I told the following story—the first story—for the first time. And wept. I wept and I wept. It was an archetypal therapy moment, right out of the playbook. Over time, I began to tell this story outside of therapy. For quite a while I could only share it with certain people, and under the right circumstances—when I sensed the appreciated gravity. The second story is reflective of the time I finally became able to tell the first as if it were just generically devastating, and not so much the definitive and shameful truth of who I am, encapsulated. But this newfound ability didn't minimize the importance of it. It's still a life-shaping story.

So anyway, when I was young, we visited my relatives every year for Thanksgiving. My family was as dysfunctional as any, and the yearly event was not all sunshine and lollipops. In fact, unlike at my doctor's office, lollipops were strictly forbidden. As the designated problem in my nuclear family, and for whatever complicated reasons, my extended family, my weight during a holiday focused on food was a convenient distraction from whatever other issues the family was avoiding. It was never a comfortable time for me, to say the least. One year, and I was far too young to know what precipitated this drama, it was decided that I was not to have pie. Dieters do not eat pie. That's simple enough, and special occasions were not an exception. Whether or not I was the only dieter in the bunch, I don't know, but I was the only dieter under the age of ten who could be singled out and ordered to be an example for all the others, who were old enough to determine if Thanksgiving was a legitimate cheat day, for them.

There were twenty-five or thirty people in the house. The table was in the dining room on the ground floor, right off the stairs. From the stairs you could see the dining room, though if a person was seated at the far end of the table, they probably couldn't see the stairs. That covered maybe a half dozen of the guests; the rest had a good view. I don't recall who exactly came up with this plan, it was probably my grandmother because this is her kind of plan, but upon the serving of the pumpkin, pecan, and mince-meat, I was asked to leave the table. Indeed, I was ordered to leave the table. I was told to sit on the stairs and watch the pie-eating ritual: I'll have pumpkin, or I'll have a sliver of each.

For reasons I will never understand, I was made to sit about halfway up the stairs. Or maybe I chose that spot. Out of pie reach, but still able to watch the consummation of the event. And twenty-five or thirty people were able to watch me watch the consummation, which I can't imagine added much to their eating enjoyment, particularly because as I sat my fat eight- or nine-year-old behind on the stairs watching, I quietly cried, the entire time. I was eight or nine years old; I wasn't crying for lack of pie, I was crying for lack of understanding. The tears of alienation. Alienation became a long-standing issue in my life. Perhaps needless to say.

As I sat on the stairs, and the pie eaters ate their pie, there was no acknowledgment of me. I can't fathom how awkward it must have been, at least for those who had any capacity for empathy. But no one, neither adult nor child, broke the mandate, which apparently included acting as if I did not exist—crying on the stairs, watching the pie eaters eat pie—a group including most of the people in the world who were supposed to love me. I guess they were supposed to protect me as well, but I find that notion dubious. At one point, either staged or not, I will never know, my uncle climbed the stairs. He stopped, patted me on the back, and said, "You are very brave." Brave? Not really. Powerless? For sure. And so very, very alone.

And that is the first story. The second story is much more recent; in fact, it is in the present.

Although I did many years of talk therapy, and each time I made progress (whatever that means), my most recent experience was a very different kind of therapy. I went for what I thought was eating-disorder treatment; at least that is what the place I went to specialized in. I had been recovering, as they say, from disordered eating for years, and relatively speaking, it was pretty well under control. But I still binged, or ate emotionally, or had periods of overeating, or whatever you want to call it. And it still bothered me.

When I met the therapist and told her a bit about my history, it turned out we didn't actually focus on eating at all. Instead, she diagnosed me with post-traumatic stress disorder. Why I had never been diagnosed with that before still eludes me; it was so damn obvious. At any rate, there is a very specific technique that is often used to treat PTSD—it is called EMDR (eye movement desensitization and reprocessing), which succinctly, according to WebMD, "involves presenting the patient with various visual and tactile stimuli meant to release emotional experiences and free the mind of blockages." It's in this process (which sounds like a cross between magic and complete bullshit) that the therapist has you follow her finger (or some object) with your eyes, while you focus on a predetermined thought. The concept is that painful memories can be moved to a different part of the brain, to be stored in such a way that they become matter-of-fact, as opposed to traumatic. And this exercise of focusing on a thought while engaging in some other stimulation, like eye movement, shifts those memories to the new area in the brain, where they sit quietly minding their own business.

There have been studies of the technique with brain scans, and people who believe in it believe very strongly. I believe, because it was not only the most difficult therapy I ever engaged in but was also the most effective, without a doubt. I can't say for sure whether EMDR is the miracle some say it is, or I was just "ready" for the resolution. Nonetheless, it was an astonishing experience.

But that is not the story. The second story is this: My therapist was getting ready to go on maternity leave, and she was preparing me to either end therapy or see someone else. I felt it was time to end it, and I sure as hell didn't want to start that again with someone new. So she let me go, but not before setting me up with a kind of "safe place" in my head. Somewhere I could go emotionally when I was feeling vulnerable. Although I have been trained as a therapist myself, I can't tell you why this kind of thing works. Just accept it as part of the story. I do.

As part of this process, she asked me to describe myself as an object, and what I came up with was an amorphous blob. Before I give you more details about that, I will interject that of all the things I have discussed, all the stories I have told, this is the most private. No one knows about the amorphous blob. No one knows any of what I am about to explain. Not even my therapist, because most of it evolved after she went off to have a baby and I was on my own. I tell this very private, and perhaps peculiar story, because if I can just help just one person...blah, blah, blah. And, because if you have a fat kid they might have PTSD, and if you were a fat kid, you might have PTSD, and EMDR seems to be pretty effective for PTSD.

Anyway, I left therapy with this idea that I was an amorphous blob—not so much because I am fat, but because that is where my brain went when she asked the question. It wasn't really about fat, as much as a reflection of my perception of my existence as a whole. I can't explain it much better than that, and frankly if it doesn't matter to me, it shouldn't matter to you.

Shortly after, I separated myself, in my mind, from the amorphous blob. It became something distinct from myself. It also became the central figure I would go to when I was in trouble and needed a safe place. The actual safe location for me and the amorphous blob to hang out, in my head, was an empty room—just a generic completely empty room with bare walls and a cold floor. The amorphous blob was there to wrap me in warmth and give me shelter. If you would like to picture it, the amorphous blob is white, and it looks like a cross between a giant beanbag chair, a fluffy cloud, and taffy. Comfortable to lie on and completely malleable, the amorphous blob is also a shape-shifter.

From there, other characters emerged in my safe place. First came the tiger. The tiger is what you imagine a tiger to be, though it is a particularly majestic tiger. Beautiful and proud and completely fearless at its job, which is to protect me from whatever I need protecting. The tiger is my sentry and the guardian of my safe place. The tiger is proud of its work. The tiger is fierce to its foes, but always gentle to those permitted in my safe place.

Along with me, the amorphous blob, and the tiger, came my dog. My actual dog, though just in my mind. My dog is Ella and her role in all of this is to be my dog. She gets to be in the safe place with me because of unconditional love, and because I would never go anywhere like a safe place without her. Somewhere along the road, a baby doll showed up. It's a baby doll—like a fake baby. I've come to realize that the baby doll is me, but not yet in living form. I'll be ready to take on her identity when I'm ready. Do your own analysis of that one; it's pretty straightforward. And then the final member of the brigade is the monster.

To be clear on how this all works in my head, Monster, and all of these players are referred to by their proper names: Monster, Tiger, The Baby, and Amorphous Blob. I am just me and Ella is just Ella.

Monster came along considerably later. At first Monster wasn't allowed in the safe place, or more specifically the safe room. We would watch him through a large pane of glass. Monster is a he; I can't tell you why. Monster represented binge eating, as it was originally my theoretical contention that Monster was the one doing all the binge eating. It was Monster who became out of control and dangerous to me. And that is why Monster wasn't allowed in the safe room. He was relegated to the outside, alienated.

Then one day while I was listening to the Rolling Stones and dancing around my house, which I do sometimes, I began to cry. Mind you, this was a couple of years ago; I was in my mid-forties. I realized I had to let Monster in the room, and that I shouldn't be mad at Monster because Monster had been protecting me too, all along. Monster was the one who found a way to cope, and the fact that Monster coped with food was not a monstrous thing, but rather a clever mechanism for survival. So, I had to forgive Monster. Monster, by the way, is a looming jet-black creature. He is made of paper, but not solid paper. He is peppered with the small cutouts of a paper snowflake, so you can see through him and although he is a monster, he is beautiful. He has always been that way. And it's not like I gave his appearance a lot of thought; that is just how he appeared when it happened.

So, crying and listening to the Rolling Stones, I opened the door to the safe room and let Monster in. Upon which, Monster and I danced. When we danced, I forgave him. And when I forgave him, he was awarded the protection of Tiger, and the comfort of Amorphous Blob, he became the primary caretaker of The Baby, and gets to be loved by Ella, unconditionally.

Of course I realized, in case you didn't see it coming: I am Monster. The monster is me.

I am not suggesting that dancing with your monster isn't a deeply life-affirming experience. I am not saying that realizing the amorphous blob is separate from yourself isn't a powerful recognition. Or that having a tiger to protect you isn't an excellent decision in positive self-care. I am not even stating that the process, however long it takes, of allowing yourself to become the baby doll isn't a worthwhile endeavor. Or that bringing your dog to the safe place isn't a superb idea. But I am saying that being a fat kid is why I have to do all of that. Actually, I'm not saying that at all. I don't have to do all of that because I was a fat kid—it's because as a fat kid I was taught to feel the world was unsafe. There are, in fact, other options.

No matter what the intentions of the first lady or my first-grade teacher, being singled out as a fat kid rather than just a kid had serious consequences. And whether you like it or not, that's the truth.

I may have a safe place but I don't have a crystal ball, so I can't say what my life would have been like if that doctor didn't put me on my first diet at six. But I can tell you that if I hadn't sat on those stairs during Thanksgiving because I was on diet, and kids on diets don't eat pie, things would have been different for me.

The moral is: A fat kid is just a kid who is fat.

> *I am he, as you are he, and you are me, and we are all together.*
> *See how they run, like pigs from a gun.*
> *See how they fly.*
> *I'm crying.*

> —"I Am The Walrus," the Beatles

ABOUT THE AUTHOR

Rebecca Jane Weinstein is the author of three books, including *Fat Sex: The Naked Truth*, part of the Fat Books series. She has also written for numerous national publications. Rebecca is the founder of PeopleOfSize.com, an online community and social networking site which provides information, support, and interaction for "people of size." An attorney and social worker with a master's degree focusing on clinical therapy, Rebecca has been working as an advocate and writer for nearly twenty years. She is considered an expert on the subject matter of weight and culture. Rebecca shares her own experiences of being a fat child, and now a fat adult, having been put on her first diet at age six. She understands the struggles that so many experience living in a world with a "war on fat." More information can be found at RebeccaJaneWeinsteinWriter.com.